Early Childhood Intervention

Early Childhood Intervention: Shaping the Future for Children with Special Needs and Their Families

Volume 1: Contemporary Policy and Practices Landscape

Volume 2: Proven and Promising Practices

Volume 3: Emerging Trends in Research and Practice

Early Childhood Intervention

Shaping the Future for Children with Special Needs and Their Families

Volume 3

Emerging Trends in Research and Practice

Louise A. Kaczmarek
Editor

Christina Groark, set editor

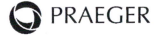 PRAEGER

AN IMPRINT OF ABC-CLIO, LLC
Santa Barbara, California • Denver, Colorado • Oxford, England

Northwest State Community College

Copyright 2011 by Christina Groark, Steven Eidelman, Louise A. Kaczmarek, and
Susan P. Maude

Library of Congress Cataloging-in-Publication Data

Early childhood intervention : shaping the future for children with special needs and their
families / Christina Groark, set editor.
    p. cm.
  Includes bibliographical references and index.
  ISBN 978–0–313–37793–8 (hard copy : alk. paper) — ISBN 978–0–313–37794–5 (ebook)
  1. Children with disabilities–Education (Preschool)—United States. 2. Children with
disabilities—Services for—United States. 3. Child development—United States. 4. Child
welfare—United States. I. Groark, Christina J.
LC4019.2.E25   2011
371.9–dc22   2011011997

ISBN: 978–0–313–37793–8
EISBN: 978–0–313–37794–5

15 14 13 12 11   1 2 3 4 5

This book is also available on the World Wide Web as an eBook.
Visit www.abc-clio.com for details.

Praeger
An Imprint of ABC-CLIO, LLC

ABC-CLIO, LLC
130 Cremona Drive, P.O. Box 1911
Santa Barbara, California 93116-1911

This book is printed on acid-free paper (∞)

Manufactured in the United States of America

For Paul, my son, and all children with special needs who deserve the best start in life that society in general, policy makers, professionals, and families can give them, and to those who advocate for them, thank you.

Contents

Preface and Acknowledgments

This series of three volumes is about special services known as *early intervention* or *early childhood special education* (EI/ECSE) provided to young children with special needs and their families. As the terms imply, these services provide support early in a child's life, even as early as birth, until the age of school entry. Specifically, early intervention as found in Part C of the IDEA 2004 Statute (P.L. 108-446) is defined as health, educational, and/or therapeutic services that are provided under public supervision and are designed to meet the developmental needs of an infant or toddler who has a developmental delay or a disability. At the discretion of each state, services can also be provided to children who are considered to be *at risk* of developing substantial delays if services are not provided. These services must be provided by qualified personnel and, to the maximum extent appropriate, must be provided in natural environments including the home and community settings in which children without disabilities participate. Early childhood special education (ECSE), as found in Part B, Section 619 of the IDEA, intends for smooth transition of a child from EI to ECSE. It stipulates that the local education agency will participate in the transition planning of a child from early intervention (Part C) to early childhood special education for a preschool-aged child the year she turns 3 years of age. The child may receive all the early intervention services listed on her service plan until her third birthday. Then she must be assessed as eligible for ECSE services

Why is this field important? First, it is scientifically known that early childhood is a time of significant brain development and substantial growth in every domain of all children's development. Second, it is widely accepted that at this time, all learning takes place in the context of relationships, and that families are central to these relationships. Therefore, for better child outcomes, short and long term, families must be involved at all levels. Third, professionals serving eligible children and families must be on the same page with the families, the children, and each other by coordinating their work and being focused on the skills that are important in the individual child's life. Fourth, this field is important because it demonstrates a connection between instruction and developmental outcomes that benefit children with or without disabilities. For example, the design of certain curricula, individualized educational programs, universal design for environments, tiered teaching methods, and other practices in these volumes are good strategies for all children, not only those with special needs.

But why attend to this particular population of children and families here and now? The prevalence of children with special needs worldwide as well as nationally is increasing. In 1991–1992, the prevalence of children with disabilities in the United States was estimated at 5.75 percent (http://www.cdc.gov/mmwr/PDF/wk/mm4433.pdf). In a more recent review (*Pediatrics* [2008], *121*, e1503–e1509) by Rosenberg, Zhang, and Robinson, the prevalence of developmental delays of children born in the United States in 2001 and eligible for Part C early intervention was indicated at 13 percent.

This growing prevalence also points to economic and public health concerns. Developmental delay, when attended to appropriately earlier in life, is shown to be lessened and thereby alleviate costs to the public. Typically, the estimated lifetime cost for those born in 2000 with a developmental disability is expected to total (based on 2003 dollars) $51.2 billion for people with intellectual disabilities, $11.5 billion for people with cerebral palsy, $2.1 billion for people who are deaf or have hearing loss, and $2.5 billion for people with vision impairment (http://www.cdc.gov/ncbddd/dd/ddsurv.htm). Early services work to significantly reduce these costs.

Also, as society, the economy, and all aspects of life are becoming more globally interdependent, it is our responsibility to help all children reach their potentials and contribute positively to our future. Our society needs a trained, talented, and diverse workforce. We cannot afford to lose the potential of such an important and large sector of children.

In addition to growing prevalence and the need for a diverse workforce, special needs affect all types of families. There is no culture, ethnic group, gender, geographic area, or socioeconomic status group that does not include children with special needs. Special needs and disabilities are inordinately diverse in terms of diagnosis, variability within a diagnosis, intensity, spectrum of characteristics, age of impact, multiplicity, and combinations of disabilities. Further, all children, typically developing or not, need some individualized attention, instruction, and care. They are not little adults. They learn by different styles and at different rates.

Because of this diversity and the importance of the development of this cohort of children, the editors worked diligently to be sure that the most current and best available research is combined with professional experiences, wisdom, and values; clinical expertise; and family-child perspectives. Although no rock was left unturned in the selection of topics and contributors, there was some difficulty in selecting topics. The advisors, editors, and publishers felt strongly that this series is to be of utility to a variety of professionals, parents, practitioners, policy makers, service trainers, students, academics, and scholars, including those not directly related to this field (e.g., a lawyer who is interested in policy, a parent who wants to know about the best supports for her child). Although we strongly intended to have the three volumes provide breadth to the readers, we still wanted them to be as comprehensive as possible. Once the topics were agreed upon, authors were easy to select because we invited the best in the field who could communicate the issues in an accurate, precise, and understandable way. Therefore, information was gathered from experience and scientific evidence by the best in the fields of early intervention and early childhood special education policy and law, medicine and health sciences, and education and child welfare, among others.

So the reader will find that the scope of this series is broad but still covers the critical components of early intervention and early childhood special education. It is organized into three volumes in such a way that readers can skim through each to find the areas of particular interest to them. The chapters within the three volumes are intended to answer key questions regarding how this field works. For instance, how do we identify children needing early intervention or early childhood special education and recognize them as early as possible? Where does this detection and subsequent service take place? Who works in early intervention, and what is their training? What is the families' role in all of this, and what are their rights? How does that role differ in early intervention compared to early childhood special education? Which programs, or what parts of programs, work best, and for whom? What does it cost to provide this service, and how effective is it? What are still some of the unknowns of this field (which is relatively young compared to other fields of study)?

Specifically, Volume 1, *Contemporary Policy and Practices Landscape*, begins with a historical perspective of this field. It then relates state policies and various attempts to implement them and international laws and sample country responses to the care, education, and development of children with disabilities. This volume also considers who provides these services; their training, background, and experiences; and evaluation of programs for quality and cost-effectiveness. Policies regarding children with special needs nationally and internationally tell us the rights of children and families. Sometimes they even tell us what should be provided and when. However, they do not tell us *how* to implement quality programs; thus, the need for Volume 2.

You will see, therefore, that the chapters in Volume 2, *Proven and Promising Practices in Early Intervention/Early Childhood Special Education*, cover the best available practices that are currently used and studied throughout the field of early intervention. These chapters include information on programs such as Early Head Start and Head Start and new, exciting model strategies and techniques in intervening with children with challenging behaviors, mental health diagnoses, sensory processing, and others. We were fortunate to find the best professionals in the fields of early intervention and early childhood special education, including individuals from occupational therapy, speech and language pathology, psychology, policy development, technology use with children, early literacy and math, teacher education, English-language learning, and specialists in visual and hearing impairments. Yet there is always room for new knowledge and improvement. That is what we hope we captured in Volume 3.

Volume 3, *Emerging Trends in Research and Practice*, creatively takes the reader into the realm of possibilities. It helps the reader think about needs of expanding or emerging populations such as culturally and linguistically diverse families and the need for schools to be prepared for learners with a wide range of needs and abilities. This volume also invites reflection on issues that are not totally resolved, like crossing systems in the delivery of services, how do we get over the financial and administrative silos in these public systems, and how do we get professionals and bureaucrats to work together to cross these systems? However, this volume also provides solutions to current issues that should be considered, advocated for, or debated, such as the Recognition and Response tiered model of instruction.

Finally, the chapters in Volume 3 point us in the direction of future research and trials of models and strategies. For instance, we need to make the best use of technology and research-based practices. Another example includes child progress monitoring and accountability. Monitoring and accountability have evolved over the years, and better practices actually may include simpler procedures. But are we capturing the complexities of teaching and learning? Do we really understand the needs of children with special needs and how to best engage their families and integrate a variety of professional recommendations for the most effective program? Finding these answers will demand a lot from professionals (e.g., to follow professional practices such as DEC-NAEYC), from researchers (e.g., to develop and test evidenced based practices), and from the public in general (e.g., to advocate).

All three volumes contain special features like matrices, graphs, and diagrams to stimulate readers not only in what is, but in what could be. They are different from other works in that they provide the state of the art in the field while considering the antecedents and the future prospective in the field. They are intended to be appealing to anyone interested in children, especially children with special needs, and to provide enough information to continue and grow that interest.

* * *

I would like to thank many people for their contributions to the creation, writing, editing, and production of this series. First, the volume editors, Steven Eidelman, Susan P. Maude, and Louise A. Kaczmarek, all of whom are first-rate professionals, child advocates, and early interventionists whom I relied upon heavily for chapter ideas, finding the best authors in the field, volume editing, writing chapters for the volumes, and fabulous contributions to the entire enterprise. There would be no series without them.

Second, my assistants, Mary Ellen Colella, Amy Gee, Mary Louise Kaminski, and Kaitlin Moore, who kept me organized, edited me and reedited me, and checked details when I could no longer see the trees through the forest.

In addition, thank you to our illustrious advisers. They came from so many different professions with the highest level of understanding of the nature of the children in these services and of what is needed by our readers. I appreciate their willingness to share their expertise openly and candidly.

And to my students, Amber Harris-Fillius, Claudia Ovalle-Ramirez, Robin Sweitzer, and Wen Chi Wang, thank you for their thorough reviews of the chapters. I learned a lot from them.

Finally, thank you to my family: Brian, Patti, Stephanie, and Paul, for teaching me about children and families and for their patience and encouragement throughout this work.

Chapter 1

Partnerships with Families from Diverse Cultures

Susan M. Moore, Clara Pérez-Méndez,
and Louise A. Kaczmarek

Box 1.1

There exists no generic entity which may be dubbed the Southeast Asian family, the Native American family . . . each of these categories encompasses numerous cultures, and their individual members may share tendencies in some areas and not in others. Individuals and families will be found to lie along different points of their cultural continuum (from traditional, for example to fully bicultural). These are valid cultural distinctions only in the very broadest sense of the term.

Anderson & Fenichel (1989)

A FAMILY STORY

"**M**y name is Marta C. My parents are Mexicans. We come from a family of two languages. As young children we spoke Spanish at home and as adults we decided to change our culture a little bit and now some of us speak English. But my culture is still Hispanic. My school was in Mexico and it was all in Spanish. I was raised in a mining town with about 500 families. We all knew each other. It was a town with lots of traditions. I have six brothers. They all had the opportunity to go out of town to go to school and the University. I was the little one and my dad couldn't afford to give me an education, so I left school. When I was 18, we moved to

Camargo, Chihuahua. I started working there. My grandmother was a United States citizen, but she never had her papers in order, because since she was a baby her father brought her to live in Mexico. She decided to get her United States citizenship papers and benefits in order. She was successful and then all her children were able to apply for citizenship. We all wanted to be together, first my uncle and his family, then my aunt and her family, and then my mother and me and my brothers, and that is how we all immigrated until we established our family here.

"Life in the U.S. for me has been very good. Here is where my life has changed completely. I can, I want, and I will do more with my life; I will improve more. I want to speak English at 100 percent. I have two children. My daughter is 8 years old and my son will be 5 years old in February and we are living in two cultures, the American and the Mexican. My husband is American. We are combining both cultures; we don't want to lose either one. We speak Spanish and English at home. If my husband says the colors in English, I say them in Spanish. When my daughter was 2 years old, she was able to say everything. When my son, Mac, was 2, he didn't. He only pointed to things and used gestures. So I was very worried about what was happening with him. We made an appointment with his pediatrician and he did a checkup. He told us that he was fine. He told us it will take him longer to talk because of the two languages, but he said he was fine. I said to myself that I couldn't be sitting and waiting years for him to talk. I couldn't as a mother just wait. I didn't believe that. The doctor said he may not have any problems, but I felt the need to do something and to look for information. I needed to find help, but who could help me?

Since I was not satisfied to wait, I made many phone calls. I finally called the Child Find at the school district. They gave me an appointment right away. This is when I realized that they spoke my language. They told me in Spanish that at this time, on this date, they will come to your house to have an interview and see about the next steps for your son. They told me that the speech-language pathologist was bilingual and would be a translator for the other professionals who were coming. I thought how perfect that they speak my language. How else could I talk to them since I didn't speak good English, if they didn't speak Spanish? My English was very minimal at this time. They introduced themselves and we talked in Spanish. They asked me lots of questions and did paperwork and then they said they didn't see any problems but they would do an evaluation in Spanish just to be sure. For us, that was the support we needed. They gave us information and suggestions on how we could help him to support his language in both Spanish and English. In the end, Mac didn't need individual therapy. He just participated in El Grupo de Familias (a university-based parent education and support group for families who speak Spanish) with me. When in El Grupo, he started participating more with other children; he started doing the things the other children were doing. He might have known how to do it before, but he felt confident to do more and express more his needs. We noticed that in him and we started using the strategies from El Grupo de Familias, here at home, and now we give him more time and find more time for him. It really has worked for us. Since he has been part of El Grupo, he is talking more and talking in both languages. That was the support he needed; he is a very healthy and intelligent boy.

"In the Hispanic community the language is the biggest barrier. Sometimes we have the information in our hands, but we are fearful to make a phone call because we don't know the English language. We think, 'what can I do if they answer in English?' People hang up. After my experience with my son, some of my neighbors asked me how did I get information. I told them not to wait, but get information now.

"After El Grupo, Mac was in preschool the next year and we were asked if we could give permission to do a screening on him. We gave our permission. That school is English only. They don't have a bilingual staff. And when the results of the test were given to us, they said that he had problems with his hearing and with his language development. I went back to the Child Find and asked if they could help me with these findings. I asked for help again and they said 'yes.' They did another hearing test, a vision test, and a lot more language tests, but this time they tested him in both Spanish and English according to the education laws. We also had an interview with them and they asked us lots of questions about his use of English and Spanish at home. They went to Mac's school and observed him one day. They decided that everything was OK again, but say his Spanish is better than his English. But it was a warning for me again! I asked, 'What is happening? Am I aware of what Mac needs?' The problem was that his school was not bilingual and the teachers didn't know that he was bilingual. He wasn't using his English or Spanish in school. Now in his new school, it's clear for the teachers that Dad is American and speaks English and Mom is Mexican and speaks Spanish and both languages are spoken at home. The bilingual speech-language pathologist who tested Mac at Child Find and observed him in his school stopped by Mac's school to give the teachers some suggestions about how to help Mac use his English more and how to help him feel more confident and comfortable speaking English. Mac speaks more Spanish, but he is trying to speak more English too, and he says, 'I speak English and Spanish,' and he says this with a lot of pride."

LEARNING FROM FAMILY STORIES

What is important about Marta's story? What worked for Marta in her interactions with teachers, professionals, and other resources? What was concerning about her story? How would you respond to her concerns and situation?

Because language and culture are so interdependent, communicating with families from different cultural and linguistic backgrounds can be very complex. When the language of the family and the provider are different, it is clear that communication can be severely compromised. However, speaking the same language does not guarantee communication. Lynch and Hanson (2004) remind us that communication, both verbal and nonverbal, is critical to developing partnerships with families. By taking the time to develop relationships and truly listen to family stories, their concerns, and their priorities, early interventionists and related specialists can understand families' past and present experiences, identify family strengths and resilience, and encourage the establishment of meaningful relationships by understanding the interaction between language and culture in the lives of families (Bruns & Corso, 2001; Moore & Pérez-Méndez, 2006; Sánchez, 1999a). It is important that educators learn about the myriad factors that influence families. These include family structure, personal characteristics, citizenship, length of time since immigration, levels of acculturation and/or assimilation, languages spoken by the family, and most importantly, cultural expectations for their children, early childhood education, and early intervention services. It is critical in this process of listening to families that early childhood educators and providers of services remember that all families vary in the degree in which their beliefs and life ways may represent a particular culture, language group, religious group, or country of origin (Anderson & Fenichel, 1989; Moore & Pérez-Méndez, 2006; Thorp, 1997). To develop authentic relationships with educators and other professionals, family perspectives need to be heard and acknowledged. Families need to feel listened to and trust that early childhood interventionists and professionals have their children's best interest in mind. Knowledge, skills, and attitudes of educators and other professionals need to be

---

Box 1.2

What they need . . . they need to know about our culture . . . how we raise our kids . . . what we do when they are sick . . . when they are with adults . . . when they eat, and when they go to school. They need to learn how we think and feel as a family about our kids.

—Maria Sandoval, Parent

To make progress and have a family go in a positive direction, the family has to feel valued . . . that the information they are sharing is just as important as is the information the professionals are sharing . . . for the family to feel this is critical to success.

—Linda Roan Yager, Parent

---

developed to fully address the often complicated issues and circumstances surrounding the education of our youngest and most vulnerable learners, especially those that also have disabilities.

The purpose of this chapter is to explore the concepts of family-centered, culturally competent, and responsive practices that build reciprocal relationships and strengthen partnerships with diverse families in the delivery of early intervention services.

CHANGING WORLD

The rapid growth of our youngest population challenges our present support system for meeting the needs of children and their families who may be culturally and/or linguistically diverse, especially those receiving early intervention services or those at risk for disabilities. The demographic profile of our earliest learners is changing dramatically as we strive to address the developmental and early education needs of our early childhood population generally and to meet the very specific needs of such children with diagnosed disabilities. The PEW Research Center (Passel & Cohn, 2008) projects the racial and ethnic mix of our population will look quite different in 2050, with a significant increase in the Hispanic and Asian populations. By 2050, it is projected that one in four children in the United States will be of Hispanic origin (Forum on Child and Family Statistics, 2010). It is important to consider that 77 percent of children who enter public school coming from non-English-speaking homes speak Spanish, with the next two highest groups being Vietnamese (2.4%) and Hmong (1.8%; Keller-Allen, 2006). However, 325–341 different languages are spoken or represented in the population of the United States and nearly 6 percent of the U.S. population either does not speak English or does not speak English well (Hernandez, 2004; Capps, Michael, Ost, Reardon-Anderson, & Passel, 2004).

UNDERSTANDING THE EVOLVING CONCEPT OF FAMILY THROUGH A CULTURAL LENS

Families are described as "big, extended, nuclear, multi-generational, with one parent, two parents, and grandparents. We live under one roof or many. A family can be as temporary as a few weeks, or as permanent as forever. We become part of a family by birth, adoption, marriage, or from a desire for mutual support. A family is a creature unto itself, with different values and unique ways of realizing its dreams; together our families become the source of our rich cultural heritage and spiritual diversity . . . our families create neighborhoods, communities, states, and nations" (Report from the House Memorial 5 Task Force on Young Children and Families, New Mexico, 1990, p. 2). Every one brings their own culture, values, beliefs, and experiences to each relationship that is developed with a family during the delivery of early intervention services. Background and experiences affect everything one does and provides a "cultural lens" through which we view how children are raised, how households are organized, how one talks, what languages are spoken, how disability is viewed, and how education is viewed. Unfortunately, individuals may not be aware of the impact of culture on their behaviors, habits, and customs (Hall, 1976). Given this breadth and depth of diversity, early intervention professionals need to adjust their cultural lens to "wide angle" to understand others' experiences, values, and beliefs and how these influence each and every family. This understanding, which unfolds as the relationship progresses, provides the foundation from which family-professional partnerships are developed and sustained.

Perspectives on Culture: A Continuum

Anderson and Fenichel (1989) conceptualize culture as a "specific framework of meanings within which a population, individually and as a group, shapes it life ways (p. 1)." The way of life of a group of people includes shared values, beliefs, world views, social reality, roles and relationships, and patterns or standards of behavior (such as communication style, child rearing practices, and family composition). These dimensions of culture often describe features with which an individual may identify.

Although many link cultural features to a sense of shared ancestry and continuity with the past, others may base them upon factors of race, ethnicity, nationality, and geographic locations. However, it is also important to consider other dimensions when describing diversity (Chen, Brekken, & Chan, 1998). Dimensions of culture as described by Sánchez and Thorp (2008) include those that are readily recognizable or "tangible," like dress, food, holidays and artifacts. They contrast tangible aspects to those that are "intangible" and sometimes more difficult to recognize. Yet, they note that in their research and experience, the intangible aspects of culture more powerfully impact interactions among early childhood educators and interventionists, other professionals, children, and family members. These may include deeply held beliefs and traditions about child rearing, appropriate ways for children to interact with adults, play, feeding patterns, and ways to discipline young children. Differences in beliefs between family and professionals can provide fertile ground for cultural conflicts necessitating dialogue and resolution. Lynch and Hanson (2004) offer a set of continua representing other "intangible" values and beliefs, which are particularly relevant to working with families within early intervention. These include the continua of extended family on one end, to the nuclear family on the other; interdependence to individuality; nurturance to independence; tradition to technology; broad ownership to individual/specific ownership; differentiated rights to equal rights; and harmony to control.

Culture is understood by many to be a dynamic, ongoing process, within which individuals are constantly revising or trying out new ideas and behaviors that fit their life ways. According to Lynch and Hanson (2004), culture is not static, but rather dynamic and everchanging. These authors point out that when describing any culture or cultural practice, *within group differences* are as great if not greater than *across group differences*. Within group heterogeneity is influenced by many factors, yet when terms such as *cultural identity, differences*, or *diversity* are used, it is important to recognize that dimensions of culture and ethnicity are typically framed in terms of differences in relation to another group, most typically the majority/mainstream culture. This is a critical consideration if early interventionists are to widen their "cultural lens" and acknowledge their own beliefs, values, and biases that impact their work with families. Many authors (Hall, 1976; Harry, Kalyanpur, & Day, 1999; Lynch & Hanson, 2004; Moore & Pérez-Méndez, 2003; Sánchez & Thorp, 2008) suggest it is imperative to recognize that each and every person is a product of one or more cultures. Chen and colleagues (1998) describe the concept of cultural assumptions as being beliefs that are so completely accepted within a group that they do not need to be recognized explicitly or questioned. However, there is danger in assuming that because a family has certain cultural beliefs in common, they can be stereotyped in terms of adhering to all beliefs and patterns associated with their culture (Moore & Pérez-Méndez, 2006). Each and every family deserves *individual consideration* regardless of cultural identity. Faulty assumptions, when working with families from cultures different from one's own, can be at the root of misunderstandings and conflicts, such as how young children are disciplined or the role of professionals in the development of young children. Assumptions that lead to conflict can often be successfully avoided or resolved through adoption of a "wide angle" cultural lens—that is, the basic understanding of dimensions of culture and the development of a relationship with each and every family characterized by mutual communication and information sharing.

Perspectives on Assimilation and Acculturation

An understanding of the concepts of assimilation and acculturation are basic to recognizing how culture is dynamic and ever changing. The term assimilation is often used to describe identified groups who give up their culture and adopt the common values and beliefs of a mainstream culture. Assimilation can be forced (e.g., indigenous cultures/tribal groups) or, for many immigrant populations, a reaction to fear of discrimination and prejudice. However, it can also be a choice by those wanting to adopt the life ways of the majority culture, a choice often ascribed to those immigrants coming to the United States to avoid war or religious or political persecution.

Acculturation, in contrast, is a process often considered along a continuum, describing those who hold fast to their traditional life ways and beliefs on one side to those who not only operate primarily within the dominant culture, but also adopt its standard values. Families may move about on this continuum, often associated with choice (e.g., bicultural and bilingual) to maintain aspects of cultural identity while adopting aspects of the mainstream or dominant culture. This conceptualization of acculturation demands that one understands that family stories are not stagnant, or a set of experiences frozen in time (Moore & Pérez-Méndez, 2006; Sánchez & Thorp, 2008; Sánchez, 1999a). For example, many immigrants who have entered this country have given up their culture, language, and prior life ways in attempts to achieve success, based upon the belief that this is what is necessary for themselves and their children to succeed. Other families may retain their native language and traditions while acquiring a new language and adopting life ways similar to the mainstream culture to achieve what they consider to be success. Changes may be made while maintaining key connections to families of origin, including the ability to communicate through their first or home language, and to maintain their self-identity, culture, and self-esteem. In a pluralistic society, many individuals recognize the benefits of maintaining their own cultures of heritage while adopting newly formed life ways and beliefs.

HOME LANGUAGE AND CULTURE

Learning More than One Language

Unfortunately, it is still common that many early interventionists believe that learning a second language is most successful when the first language is abandoned or given up. They then advise parents to stop talking to their children in their heritage language, even when family members are not proficient in English, because their young children enter early education settings and are learning English. Persistence of this "myth" or misperception (Espinosa, 2008; Moore & Pérez-Méndez, 2006) about how children learn languages often creates a conundrum for those families who value their first language and want their young children to become bilingual, thus sustaining their cultural and linguistic identity. Parents often seem confused and frustrated about what languages their child should learn to be successful in school and in life, especially given family priorities to maintain communication with extended family members and maintain aspects of culture. Parents report "losing a language is like losing a world".

(Pérez Méndez & Moore, 2004). Families and their children may feel disenfranchised, misunderstood, or discriminated against when the first language is essentially devalued (Moore & Pérez-Méndez, 2006; Sánchez & Thorp, 2008; Wong Fillmore, 1991). Many families come from a background or have had prior experiences of prejudice and discrimination based upon their spoken language or even their name. Young children may also experience feelings of isolation and marginalization related to devaluing of their home language and culture (Sánchez & Thorp, 2008).

There is emerging research that suggests eliminating first languages actually results in lowered performance in overall learning and academics (Espinosa, 2008; Genesee, 2008; Sánchez & Thorp, 2008). Current research also speaks to the cognitive, social, academic, and economic advantages of bilingualism (August & Hakuta, 1997; Bialystok, 2001; Genesee, Paradis, & Crago, 2004; Hakuta, 1986; Lindholm-Leary, 2005; Lindholm-Leary & Borsato, 2006; Yoshida, 2008). Growing evidence implies that maintaining home language regardless of disability may strengthen a child's ability to transfer knowledge to learning a second language, while enhancing connections to culture and heritage and communication with family, as well as establishing a strong self-identity (Espinosa, 2008; Genesee, Paradis, & Crago, 2004; Kohnert, Yim, Nett, Kan, & Duran, 2005; Pérez-Méndez & Moore, 2004; Restrepo et al., 2010; Winsler, Diaz., Espinosa, & Rodriguez, 1999). Updated research tells us all children are capable of learning more than one language. Just because a child has a challenge or disability, it cannot be automatically assumed that he or she cannot learn two languages (Genesee, 2008; Genesee, Paradis & Crago, 2004; Kohnert, 2008; Tabors, 2008).

For many families, language learning is more than learning a language for academic success. It is also important to recognize the impacts of language learning as interdependent and developed within a cultural context. The primary cultural environment for young children is the immediate and extended family (Moore & Pérez-Méndez, 2003, 2006; NAEYC, 1995; van Kleeck, 1994). Language is the major vehicle within the family for communicating values and expectations, expressing care and concern, providing structure and discipline, and interpreting world experiences. According to Kohnert, Yim, Nett, Kan, and Duran (2005), it is critical that young children and their primary care providers share a common language, and if it is developed to the greatest degree possible, the shared language can become the foundation for continued meaningful interpersonal communication within the family throughout the child's life.

Sociohistorical Influences on Language and Culture

Clearly the timing of sociopolitical challenges, strife, and wars in our history as a country have significantly influenced patterns of language use and maintenance among various indigenous and immigrant populations. For example, parents of young children of Latino heritage speak of the discrimination of segregated schools that their own parents endured when growing up before and during the 1960s in many parts of the country. This in turn led to a significant loss of the Spanish language within the next generation, given parental fear of discrimination and prejudice against their children (Pérez-Méndez & Moore, 2004; Sánchez, 1999).

Similarly, Native Americans in the nineteenth century were the target of a concerted effort by the American government for assimilation through educational reform when young children were forced to attend residential schools away from the reservation, discouraging all traditional life ways. Children were punished for speaking their heritage language. Historical chronicles and stories of separation of young children from their families on Indian reservations also significantly impacted the numbers of primary language speakers remaining in Native American tribes across the country. According to Darrell Kipp (2007), a Blackfeet linguist, poet, and teacher, the notion of reviving the Blackfeet language was met by hostility by his tribal members when he first began to revitalize the language in preschools and later elementary school during the 1980s. He notes that it was not until 1990 that Congress passed a Native American language bill that as least acknowledged the legality of speaking tribal languages. Efforts to revitalize heritage language is successfully underway in many tribal communities today as a way to reinvest and restore lost cultural and religious traditions and to develop individual self-esteem while preventing or ameliorating current trends of marginalization among the youth from these cultures.

Culturally marginal individuals are those individuals who essentially follow their own way and do not identify with any particular cultural group. In some instances, these individuals reject their culture of heritage but are not accepting of or accepted by the values and life ways of the mainstream, and thus are considered marginalized from society. A seminal article by Wong Fillmore (1991) presents reports from many families (Asian, Korean, American Indian, Arab, Latino) that as their children lost their native language proficiency for various reasons and as they developed English, their cultural identity, values, and beliefs were often put in jeopardy. Most importantly, they lost their connection to home and ability to communicate with family. Wong Fillmore (1991) attributed this to a society that did not value multiculturalism.

Interpersonal Impact of Language Loss

Stories and reports abound in which language loss within families can compromise parent-child attachment, result in less communication, and decrease family cohesion. It is considered critically important by many authors for young children to learn the languages of their parents, who then can take full responsibility for socializing them and preparing them for schooling later on. Culture and language are considered the building blocks of self-identity and connection to family. Language and the associated cultural heritage are viewed as critical components of growth and development in young children. Elimination of languages may in fact lead to negative consequences of discontinuity with language and learning, disconnection with family, and disenfranchisement from community and heritage (Krashen, 1999; Nieto, 2000; Sánchez & Thorp, 2008; Tabors, 2008; Tatum, 2003; Wong Fillmore, 1991).

Losing some aspects of the first language is a possibility for children who are learning English as a second language (Genesee, Paradis, & Crago, 2004). However, the available research evidence does not convincingly support withholding exposure to English during the early childhood years (Genesee, 2008; Kohnert et al., 2005). There are differences in opinions about what is optimal timing for introducing a second language, and there are many influencing factors to be considered given there are an increasing number of children are not formally introduced to a second language of instruction until age 5 or above (Kayser, 2008; Sánchez & Thorp, 2008; Tabors, 2008). The research as yet does not provide clear answers for typically developing young children, nor is there research that addresses this question for children with diagnosed disabilities. But perhaps a more important question is, how can early interventionists and other professionals develop relationships with families that respect and support children's interactions in those languages spoken at home?

FAMILY-CENTERED, CULTURALLY COMPETENT, AND RESPONSIVE PRACTICES

What exactly does it mean when we say early interventionists need to adopt family-centered, culturally competent, and responsive practices when partnering with families of young children they serve? A thoughtful and thorough examination of these concepts is called for as most early interventionists acknowledge the need and are invested in developing positive relationships with families that contribute to the quality of programs provided. In a meta-analysis of the research regarding the concept of family-centered practices, Dunst, Trivette, and Hamby (2008) developed a comprehensive and descriptive profile of what it means to be family-centered.

> Family-centered practices are characterized by beliefs and practices that treat families with dignity and respect; provide practices that are individualized, flexible, and responsive to family situations; involve information sharing so that families can make informed decisions; provide family choice regarding any number of aspects of program practices and intervention options; build parent-professional collaboration and partnerships as a context for family-program relations; and promote the active involvement of families in mobilization of resources and supports necessary for them to care for and rear their children in ways that produces optimal child, parent, and family benefits. (p. 1)

This seems a tall order for many early educators and interventionists who may neither understand the components nor have had experience in implementing family-centered principles. Sánchez (1999a, p. 2) states, "the implementation of family centered practice often seems like an elusive goal, even when working with populations matching our own backgrounds, but is further complicated when working with culturally and linguistically diverse populations whose views and language are different from our own." It can become further complicated when one considers the concept of cultural competence and responsivity in practice, although there are obvious overlaps in these concepts and practice.

Developing Cultural Competence

Sue, Ivey, and Peterson (1996) described a stage approach to developing cultural competence. The first stage or step is development of *cultural awareness*. Cultural awareness involves a provider's sensitivity to his or her own personal beliefs, values, and biases and how they might influence perceptions of a family. The next step towards cultural competence focuses on *cultural knowledge*. Providers seek information and knowledge about the worldviews and expectations of the families with whom they are working. The third step is the development of *cultural skills*, involving the provider's ability to communicate and interact in a manner that is culturally sensitive and relevant to a family and situation.

Lynch and Hanson (2004) suggest a "transactional and situational approach" in which each child is recognized as an individual with unique characteristics, strengths, and needs. Families are recognized as having unique concerns, priorities, and resources. To work effectively with families, it is suggested that providers adjust and adapt strategies continuously with families, and that this may sometimes mean adapting to radically different and individualized values beliefs and practices that are different from their own. These authors suggest that building partnerships with families from cultures different from one's own can sometimes be frustrating and require further study and information gathering; and/or it can be an opportunity to be exposed to a richness of human experiences, to learn new information, and to grow as an individual. Regardless, early interventionists have been directed to address this challenge of developing family-centered, culturally competent, and responsive practices in their everyday interactions with families and children. The development of this "wide-angle lens" demands changes in dispositions, knowledge, and skills (Lynch & Hanson, 2004; Moore & Pérez-Méndez, 2003, 2006; Sánchez & Thorp, 2008; Westby, 2009).

DISPOSITIONS AND ATTITUDE

In terms of dispositions and attitude, a wide-angle lens requires that early interventionists working with families from cultures different from their own embark on a "personal cultural journey" as described by Lynch and Hanson (2004) and suggested by many other authors (Hepburn, 2004; Pérez-Méndez & Moore, 2004; Sánchez, 1999b). This journey involves in-depth self-reflection regarding one's own background, upbringing, history, and recognition of privilege for some and experiences and feelings that involve cultural discrimination and/or prejudice for others. Recognizing one's own cultural perspective opens up the way to discovering how every individual identifies with one or a combination of cultural beliefs, values, and life ways. Many individuals may not recognize how deeply ingrained key messages from our family of origin or our life's journey has impacted our behavior toward others. For example, Sánchez and Thorp (2008) describe the reaction of an early childhood student who, prior to engaging in a self-reflective process about her background, values, and beliefs, thought of herself as being without a culture. "I assumed I was just a regular American and that culture was something exotic, something other people have" (Sánchez & Thorp, 2008, p. 84). The journey can also lead to recognition of one's own cultural biases and how they can influence premature perceptions or assumptions about others. It can lead to an awareness of a historically *subtractive attitude* towards difference in others, attributed to a parochial society that is intolerant of those who speak a different language, hold certain beliefs or values that alienate them from the mainstream, practice a different religion, or engage in child-rearing practices that are assumed to harm a child. An outcome of the cultural journey can be to develop a broader perspective: an *additive* attitude that recognizes strengths and richness in cultural heritage, appreciates differences and life ways of others, and authentically celebrates diversity in classroom practices and connections to home. An additive attitude about differences combines with family-centered practices that assumes competence in families to make the best decisions they can about their children, when provided information and choices. This attitude precludes acting on assumptions about a parent, often associated with stereotypes related to cultural life ways, and thus demands *individual consideration* of each and every family. Development of an additive perspective about differences can lead to positive relationships with families built upon trust and respect.

Dispositions or attitudes can also be described as *responsive* versus *restrictive*. Responsive dispositions that recognize and appreciate the values and beliefs of a family drive responsive practices within early intervention services that enhance connections to home. Restrictive attitudes preclude open dialogue about differences or perspectives different from one's own or implementation of family practices or routines that could be adapted or followed within the delivery of early intervention services. Restrictive attitudes can lead to cultural clashes that are difficult to resolve, and interfere with the development of authentic parent-professional partnerships. There is a risk of isolation and alienation on the part of families who see their choices for early intervention restricted to the ways and beliefs of the dominant society. On the other hand, responsive dispositions recognize that differences in family belief systems, child-rearing practices, and modes of parent-child interaction represent important ways in which culture is embedded in a process of socialization of a child by family during the early childhood years. Different ways of caring for and teaching children at home are not automatically judged as contrary to developmentally appropriate practice. Cross-cultural differences in parental expectations for attainment of developmental milestones may be more representative of a basic value of interdependence than a problem in parenting.

Attitudes and dispositions can also be described as *dynamic* versus *static*. Just as children change over time, so do families. There is considerable variability among child-rearing practices that promote healthy development and learning, much of which is embedded in cultural practices passed on from one generation to the next. Yet these are continually transformed by each generation based upon the times and opportunities available. Culture evolves in a dynamic way that early interventionists can appreciate. Families also may change their stories as well as their expectations for their children with increased experience with educators and programs that allow for and recognize change.

Dispositions or attitudes can also be described as *open* or *closed*—open to the possibilities of new learning and changes in practice, or closed to differences as beyond the boundary of what is comfortable or can be considered. Recognition that changes in practice in the delivery of early intervention services can happen only when one is open to change. *Additive, responsive, dynamic*, and *open* dispositions toward cultural, linguistic, and ability diversity can shape what is possible in changing practices in the venues in which early intervention services are delivered. These dispositions positively impact foundational processes of building reciprocal relationships with families based on trust and respect.

Knowledge and Skills

Learning and gaining knowledge of cultures is another necessary step toward effective family-centered and culturally competent practices. There are a variety of strategies that a professional might use to assist in widening their cultural lens.

Reading Published Biographies, Memoirs, and Ethnographies

Resources that describe cultural life ways and differences abound. Personal biographies and ethnographic studies provide a rich resource for those open to learning more about differences in culture and experiences. For example, the ethnography *The Spirit Catches You and You Fall Down* (Fadiman, 1997) is a story of a Hmong family with several children who eventually immigrated to California after dislocation following the Vietnam War. Their daughter was diagnosed with a seizure disorder, and the basic lack of interpreters of this family's language led to numerous misunderstandings with the physicians and staff caring for her. In sum, absence of culturally competent and responsive practices, and mounting distrust on both sides, led to tragic and dire consequences for this child. Readers learned of the Hmong culture, including the history surrounding patterns of immigration, and traditional life ways and beliefs that conflicted with Western medical practices. As the story unfolds, readers learn consequences of ongoing misunderstandings and faulty assumptions stemming from a lack of understanding and knowledge of cultural life ways and miscommunications associated with a paucity of trained interpreters or cultural mediators to bridge the gap.

Participating in Diverse Community Activities

Learning often occurs "just in time" when new and diverse children become eligible for early intervention services. Interventionists providing services need to tap into resources that help them understand differences in cultures and what they might need to be aware of in relationship to building partnerships with individual families, to avoid biased ethnocentric value judgments, and prevent intrusive or inappropriate practices. Sánchez (1999) suggests knowledge about cultures can be actively pursued by *moving out of your comfort zone* and participating in community activities that involve people from cultures that are different from one's own, by engaging in activities that involve individuals and families that follow different traditions and life ways to gain perspective and understanding. She also speaks to ethical and professional responsibility to actively counter instances of discrimination or prejudice in the lives of children and families and intentionally advocate for fair and equitable practices in our early care and education systems.

Honing communication skills that facilitate and promote resolution of cultural conflicts through adoption of an *anchored understanding* of family perspectives based upon respect, reciprocity, and reframing of issues are described by Barrera and Corso (2003). Strategies for skilled dialogue with families often demands going to a *third space* to avoid getting stuck in either/or solutions to negatively charged conflicts. These authors advise early interventionists to reframe perceived negative statements and go to a third space to generate alternatives that clarify expectations and resolve conflicting perspectives when working with families.

Dialoguing with Families

Other effective ways to gather information involve dialogue and conversations that utilize ethnographic interviewing strategies with family members (Westby, 1990, 2009) or adapted person-centered planning strategies (Moore & Pérez-Méndez, 2003, 2006) that open up the conversation and dialogue and provide a framework for parents and family members to actively share information and participate in planning programs for their child. *Pathways: A Child and Family Journey* (CLC, 1992), is one example of an individualized planning process that can lead to a richer, deeper understanding of a child you work with, including:

- The family's perspective about their child
- Family expectations, questions, priorities, resources, and supports
- A profile or description of the child's strengths, style of learning, frustrations, and individual characteristics

The process is intended to be used with families as a guide to sharing valuable information with early interventionists, providers, teams, and anyone else the family chooses to participate. The framework individualizes the planning process for each child and family's journey in the context of culture and community. In this process, parents are first encouraged to share words that describe their child. "Who is Carmen?" "What words come to mind when you think about her?" This allows parents to share the strengths they see in their child and sets the tone for early interventionists to listen to descriptions of a child based on their strengths versus their deficits. Other questions are provided to continue the conversation as needed; however, the tool is typically used as a way to record parental perspectives about their child, what they like to do, how they learn, what is hard and frustrating for them, and the key questions that parents may have related to their child's educational plan. Use of this tool allows parents and family members to lead the conversation and share relevant information that can be used to understand the child in the context of their family. The process explores ways to recognize and build upon family and child strengths to promote participatory interactions and utilizes practical everyday activities, routines, and relationships to enhance child development at home, in school, and in community. *Pathways* creates an ongoing process for documenting the growth and development of the child and is easily adapted for use with all families including those who speak a language other than English (see Figure 1.1).

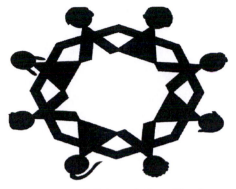

<u>Pathways: A Child and Family Journey</u> ©

Pathways: A Team's Journey provides an interactive record of your team's dialogue and reflections that begin their team-based planning process for change. As "best practice" evolves in early intervention, teams need to continually reinvent themselves as they reflect on ways to improve supports and services to young children and their families. Reciprocal information sharing and reflective practice that incorporates family feedback are key to this process.

Pathways: A Child's Journey was developed to:

- ♦ Guide families, teachers, support staff team, and anyone else the family chooses to invite, with a way of sharing valuable information.
- ♦ Individualize the planning process for each child's journey in the context of their family culture and community.
- ♦ Explore ways to use a child's and family's strengths to promote growth and development.
- ♦ Utilize practical, everyday activities and routines to enhance each child's development at home, in school, and within the community.
- ♦ Create an ongoing process for recording the growth and development of the child.

Before we get together, use the following pages to jot down some notes about your child and family that you would like to share. There are some suggestions of ideas to think about on the back page.

Figure 1.1 *Pathways:* **A process for documenting the development of a child.**

Through use of a person-centered process as adapted to families, trust between families and professionals is established through information sharing and mutual understanding, which can promote autonomy (i.e., feelings of confidence and competence in decision making) and ultimately lead families to take initiative as true partners in their child's early education and intervention (Moore & Pérez-Méndez, 2006). This sets the groundwork for family engagement, advocacy, and leadership as children progress through the educational system.

Simply listening to a family story as described by Sánchez (1999a) also creates common ground to exchange information and understand the complexities of a parent's perspective about their child. Listening to Marta's story at the beginning of this chapter revealed her strengths as a parent, including her persistence in obtaining information about her son. It also describes the actions of a family-centered, culturally responsive team effort, including a bilingual speech-language pathologist and a bilingual cultural mediator. Marta's story also illustrates concerns about erroneous results of a biased assessment process with a child who was a dual-language learner, based upon inadequate information about his family. Mac was tested only in English by this English-speaking school. The story also illustrates the positive impacts from listening to a parent's concern so that the parent can be linked to appropriate community resources for information and services.

Facilitating family stories leaves control of the direction of conversations and program planning with the family, yet, if done skillfully, allows the provider to gather appropriate information and build understanding and trust. Development of knowledge and skills in gathering information and building relationships with families involves learning how to ask genuine questions that are open-ended and leave room for storytelling and reciprocal information sharing. Families build trust in relationships when their priorities are addressed, their concerns are listened to and understood, and their resources, including their strengths, are recognized and considered. All parents benefit from respectful and trusting relationships with teachers and other early intervention providers, meaningful engagement in all aspects of the assessment processes, and educational planning for their children. Opening up the dialogue and listening so that families can share important information as well as gain information that impacts their options and choices for their children demands preparation. Honing of communication skills creates an atmosphere of exchange, focusing on parent engagement and participation, recognizing the specific needs of a particular parent, refraining from use of professional jargon, and providing information. These communication skills, coupled with those that are sensitive to challenges and recognize strengths and resilience, will enhance open dialogue with families. Use of these skills avoids and precludes premature judgments based upon prior assumptions on the part of the professional. Early interventionists report being cautious, and rightfully so, as they do not want to offend families by making assumptions about their beliefs and life ways based on self-identification with a particular culture. Simply asking families in a respectful way is often the most effective way to determine their perspective, life ways, or practices.

Dinnebeil and Rule (1994) note that families will develop and respond to early educators and professionals they trust. Core competency development in developing trusting and respectful relationships with all families is necessary, yet these relationships may develop in different ways. Some families, because of their beliefs about education and past experiences, may prefer a more formal relationship with an early intervention provider, while others may prefer an informal, friendly relationship.

Respect for the uniqueness of each family system and how it is influenced by beliefs, transitions, life ways, and languages spoken builds the foundation for increasing the ability of professionals to effectively respond to the priorities, needs, and concerns of the family, which in turn can significantly enhance the growth and education of the child. Parents are then able to engage with professionals in partnerships and actively engage in their children's early intervention program both at school and at home (Bruns & Corso, 2001; Dunst et al., 2008: Moore & Pérez-Méndez, 2003, 2006; Sánchez & Thorp, 2008; Santos, Corso, & Fowler, 2005).

Knowing the Legal Requirements

When children are referred for screening and assessment, professionals must execute these processes in accordance with the law, including the communication of sufficient information to parents so that they understand the process and can participate. The Individuals with Disabilities Education Improvement Act (2004) clearly strengthened the provisions pertaining to the referral, assessment, and identification of children with disabilities whose first language is not English, with the intention of reducing the disproportional representation of this group among special education students. Children whose home language is not English have either been over- or under-identified for special education services (Keller-Allen, 2006). The law clearly states that children cannot be identified for special education solely on the basis of *limited English proficiency*. Children must be tested using non-discriminatory, multifaceted assessment measures *administered in the language and form most likely to yield accurate information on what the student knows and can do academically, developmentally, and functionally unless this is not feasible*. For most, this means assessing the child in the home language as well as English. Testing must be administered by *trained and knowledgeable personnel,* and the assessments selected must be used for the purposes for which they were determined to be valid and reliable.

Parents also are protected under the law. Parents may not be excluded from participation in the special education process because of limited English abilities. Notifications and information about the proposed activity in the special education process must be provided to parents in their native language. Interpreters must also be provided for a parent so that they are able to understand and participate in the child's IEP meeting.

Our lack of complete understanding of second-language learning as well as the availability of appropriate instrumentation make it difficult to execute fully the provisions of the law. Most English-language proficiency tests, for example, have been standardized on monolingual native speakers (Abedi, 2006). A qualitative study (Hardin, Mereoiu, Hung, & Roach-Scott, 2009) identified additional roadblocks to implementation. This study solicited information from focus groups of parents, administrators, and teachers in an urban and rural setting to better understand current and needed practices for the referral, evaluation, and placement of preschool-aged Latino children with disabilities. The results revealed inconsistent screening and evaluation methods, such as the lack of trained test administrators and knowledgeable interpreters; the lack of strategies for ensuring parent participation, such as assuming an interpreter was not needed when parents spoke some English; the absence of professional development opportunities for professionals on test administration and second-language learning; and inconsistent or contradictory policies, such as insufficient time before having to screen, refer, and evaluate children for intervention.

Using Cultural Mediators, Interpreters, and Translators

In addition to executing legal requirements, the services of well-trained cultural mediators, interpreters, liaisons, or translators is also an effective way to obtain knowledge and develop trust with families. Many early childhood and intervention programs also now employ parent-school liaisons to increase effective connections with families. A well-trained cultural mediator or parent-school liaison does more than provide the interpretation of words spoken in conversations with families (Moore & Pérez-Méndez, 2005a, 2006). Cultural mediators or brokers are typically bilingual as well as bicultural, and can easily establish connections with families given their knowledge and experience with the culture and community shared with the family. This was the case with Marta and the Child Find team that provided her with effective early intervention supports. The Child Find team members were in concert with the cultural mediator, who in this case was also bilingual and bicultural, and able to contribute substantially to Marta's comfort level, and she was able to develop trust directly with others in the program. Effective use of cultural mediators or liaisons requires teaming with early intervention professionals as well as training and experience in working with families, especially concerning practices such as confidentiality, rights and responsibilities of families, and procedural safeguards related to services. In addition, team members not familiar with the cultural aspects can learn from the cultural mediator and increase their knowledge and skills in family-centered, culturally competent, and responsive practices when working with families from cultures different from their own.

Effective interpreters and translators must have knowledge and preparation regarding early intervention practices and processes as well as proficiency (comprehension, expression, reading, and writing) in the language of translation and English. Preparation is key. We have suggested (Moore & Pérez-Méndez, 2005a, 2005b), as have others (Chen et al., 1998), that interpreters work with professionals before the targeted event and engage in a debriefing session following it to assure accurate communication. Specific skills and helpful strategies when using translators with families are summarized in Figure 1.2.

It is important to note that different styles for translation can be used effectively for different purposes. For example, a summarization technique usually requires the translator to remember large amounts of information. The danger is that the professional may speak too fast and/or that the translator may not convey important key points. Simultaneous translation often interferes with concentration as the listeners are distracted when both the speaker and interpreter are talking at once, unless equipment suitable for this method is available. Use of this equipment can work well for large and mixed groups when one

Getting Started: Those being translated and the interpreter should discuss the following information before the translated conversation begins.

Reviewing content and terminology	The person(s) being translated and the interpreter should briefly discuss what information will be covered in the conversation and define any specific terms that may be used. The interpreter should have an opportunity to consider what terminology would be appropriate in the translated language and to ask questions for clarification.
Agreements about flow of conversation	Discuss the length of phrases the interpreter is comfortable translating at a single time and briefly practice this rhythm.
Agreements about seating arrangements	Where the interpreter sits will have an impact on the relationship that is established between those communicating. It is often preferable to have the interpreter sit or stand beside the family.
Agreements about starting conversations	Decide who will start conversations and introduce people. The interpreter will then explain that they will simply repeat in the other language what is being stated.
Confidentiality	Interpreters and families should be informed that these interactions are confidential and privacy will be respected.

Engaging in a Translated Conversation

	Ideas for those being translated	Ideas for the interpreter
Initiating conversation	Introduce yourself to the family, and make sure everyone knows who is a part of the conversation and why.	Make sure everyone understands who is in the conversation and what your role is.
Eye contact	Look at the person(s) with whom you are communicating, not the interpreter.	Look at the person(s) to whom you're translating.
Regulating the flow of conversation	Use the agreed-upon length of phrases and stop at meaningful points.	Translate completely and as accurately as possible. If you need repetition or clarification, ask.
One person speaks at a time.	Be sure to allow one person to speak at a time and to be translated before you add your comment. Agree as a group, at the beginning, to avoid side conversations.	Translate one person at a time. If necessary, ask others to pause. Ask those engaged in side conversations to repeat what they've said so that you can translate it.
Seek clarification	Check in. See if the family understands you and what it is they understand.	Recognize that participants may need to seek clarification from each other and to correct any misunderstanding or misinterpretations that may have occurred.

Moore, S. M., Eiserman, W., Pérez-Méndez, C., & Beatty, J. (1998). The Spectrum Project, UCB: Boulder.

Figure 1.2   Effective skills and strategies in translated conversations.

speaker is conveying information, such as during parent meetings or workshops. Consecutive translation is an effective way for teachers to share information in conferences. In consecutive translation, the speaker provides information, chunking it and pausing frequently for the interpreter to share the information with the family. This technique is also useful for fostering questions and dialogue with family members. An ideal situation for families would be to have an early interventionist who could speak both languages. However, the paucity of bilingual educators and professionals necessitates alternative strategies to ensure families receive and can share information in their preferred language (Moore & Pérez-Méndez, 2005b).

Sharing Research-Based Knowledge

Early interventionists working with families who speak a language other than English need to increase their research-based knowledge about how children, even those with identified disabilities (Genesee, Paradis, & Crago, 2004; Pérez-Méndez & Moore, 2004), can successfully maintain growth in their first language while learning a second language. They must be familiar with current research about bilingualism and dual-language learners and consider all background variables when providing culturally responsive early learning opportunities. Sharing this information is critically important so that families themselves can make the decision about what languages their children will learn (Pérez-Méndez & Moore, 2004). In addition, parents need an accurate assessment and description of their children's abilities if a communications and/or language challenge exists. This information is necessary to understand and to determine a profile of development, but does not automatically mean that a child cannot learn more than one language (Genesee, Paradis, & Crago, 2004; Kohnert et al., 2005; Kohnert, 2008; Moore & Pérez-Méndez, 2006; Tabors, 2008).

Early interventionists need to assume that family members are competent, and that given the appropriate information, decisions made by families are to be valued and respected, regardless of the personal beliefs of the early interventionist. This is key to building trust with families who are not only concerned about the languages their children will learn, but also how this decision could impact their children's academic success. However, this can become a very complex issue when complicated by conflicting expectations, sociopolitical and/or philosophical beliefs, and contradictions in or lack of research-based evidence.

PARENT EDUCATION AND SUPPORT

Establishing effective partnerships with diverse families also involves educating and supporting families beyond the interactions involved in the delivery of early intervention services. *El Grupo de Familias* (Moore & Pérez-Méndez, 2005c) is one example of a parent education and support model developed to build "participatory" engagement and advocacy with family members who speak a language other than English. The language spoken in this group is Spanish. A cultural mediator (bilingual and bicultural) and family resource consultant meet with families, while children and siblings play and engage in language and literacy activities with bilingual early interventionists and teachers. The model promotes inclusion of those children who are identified with challenges, as well as sharing of research-based information about how children develop languages so parents can make informed decisions about what languages their child will learn. Activities and observations are designed to support parents' understanding of children's learning through demonstration, modeling, and practice of interactive storybook-reading strategies and early language and learning activities that can be transferred to everyday routines and activities in the home.

El Grupo also promotes access to community resources through group visits to library and activation of library cards to encourage future visits. Focus is placed on navigating the system of educational supports and parent-to-parent connections. Gaining trust begins to happen during an initial activity that creates a safe environment for all the parent participants of El Grupo to share their thoughts and feelings. *The Talking Stick* is offered to parents who are asked to talk about their own childhood experiences with parents and family, their first recollections of school, and their dreams and goals for their children. It is often a very emotional and revealing exchange and sets the stage for future in-depth discussions about priorities and concerns. Over several sessions, families meet together, share stories, observe their children during play activities, and learn strategies for interactive storybook reading through videotape review and discussion. The program encourages family members to interact with professionals and advocate for their children. They learn that they can impact the responsiveness of the system of supports and services when they are knowledgeable about how this system works, and when they have enough information to select the appropriate choices for their child and family. This is one model of a parent education and support program that is family-centered, culturally resonant with and responsive to parent and family priorities and need for supports.

FACTORS INFLUENCING CULTURAL COMPETENCY

Personnel Preparation

Teacher effectiveness is one of the most salient predictors of quality and outcomes in early childhood education programs. High quality in early childhood education is identified as a basic first step for educational reform (PEW Center on the States, 2010). Current research on effects of professional development programs on classroom and intervention practices and outcomes for dual-language learners is a promising area in which to effect change (Buysse, Castro, & Peisner-Feinberg, 2010; Castro, Peisner-Feinberg, Buysse, & Gillanders, 2010; Restrepo et al., 2010). Changes in preservice and in-service personnel preparation of early interventionists are needed to ensure the development and ability of personnel to implement evidence-based practices that directly involve teaching children as well as establishing and sustaining relationships with families (Buysse et al., 2010; Maude, Catlett, Moore, Sánchez, & Thorp, 2006; NAEYC, 1995; Sánchez & Thorp, 2008; Winton, McCollum, & Catlett, 2004).

Other issues in personnel preparation are seated in the paucity of native speakers of a variety of languages in our provider workforce. The demographics and cultural characteristics and languages spoken among practicing early interventionists, educators, and other professionals presents a glaring discrepancy when viewed in context based upon the wide range and numbers of culturally and linguistically diverse children and families served. The lack of well-trained interpreters, translators, cultural mediators, or liaisons also compounds the complexity of this discrepancy as noted by Moore, Pérez-Méndez, and Boerger (2006).

Policy and Social Changes

The rapid growth of dual-language learners in education has greatly challenged our present system for educating each and every child, including those representative of social-economic and cultural diversity (Goldstein, 2004). Sheer numbers alone point to the need for increased systemic change driven by policies that address the needs of culturally and linguistically diverse learners. Concern about dispro-portionate representation in special education, marked by misidentifi-cation, under-identification, and/or over-identification of children from different cultures from the mainstream, and who speak lan-guages other than English, persist; although socioeconomic impacts cannot be discounted as a major contributing factor to this situation (Artiles & Trent, 1994; Guiberson, 2009; Ortiz & Yates, 1993). Policies implemented by the Office of Civil Rights and legislative initiatives such as the No Child Left Behind Act and the Individuals with Disabil-ities Education Act (IDEA, 2004), meant to address these challenges, have not significantly changed the trend for disproportionate repre-sentation to date (De Valenzuela, Copeland, Huaqing Qi, & Park, 2006). However, focus on early identification of children's learning abilities, needs, and progress through widespread adoption of "multi-tiered models" of instruction hold promise for each and every child receiving a developmentally appropriate education and being included at the universal level of instruction. Multitiered models have not only been adopted in K–12 education as recommended in IDEA (2004), but are now focused on preventing challenges from emerging for children in pre-K programs (Burns, Appleton, & Stehouwer, 2005; Coleman, Buysse, & Neitzel, 2006; Coleman, Roth, & West, 2009). Inclusion of each and every child regardless of diverse ability, culture, or language is a policy that has been espoused by family groups and centers for many years, and current work on promising practices to effect change in focus that includes partnerships with families within a context of community appears to be on the rise as a key component to reform educational practices.

Equity and Social Justice

Concerns surrounding disparities in access to opportunities for educa-tion for all children are reflected in the current work of many authors and projects. For example, The National Center for Culturally Respon-sive Educational Systems aims to reduce the disproportionate repre-sentation of culturally and linguistically diverse students in special education. The Equity Alliance at Arizona State University is a col-laboration that represents a set of funded programs that promote equity, access, participation and outcomes for all students. The goal for these and other projects funded through the U.S. Department of Education are focused on supporting the capacity of state and local school systems to provide high-quality, effective learning opportunities for all students and to reduce disparities in academic achievement. Many of these projects also support parent and family members to actively participate in all aspects of their child's education.

The U.S. Department of Education promotes actualization of parent-school partnerships through parent resource centers located in every state. Parent training and regional assistance centers such as the PEAK Parent Center in Colorado and the PACER Center in Minnesota support parents and family members in their quest for equity, inclusion, and quality of programs for their children with disabilities. For example, the PEAK Parent Center provides training, information and technical assistance to equip families of children from birth through age 26 with strategies to advocate successfully for their children with disabilities. All of these centers and others are members of the National Coalition for Parent Involvement in Education (http://www.ncpie.org).

Other projects such as the Center for Early Care and Education Research–Dual Language Learners (CECER-DLL), housed at the Frank Porter Graham Child Development Center in North Carolina, focuses on the disparity between evidence and research-based practices versus actual practices in early care and education. Clearly, there is a present and persistent concern about equity and social justice for all children in education, including access and equity in early care and education settings. Efforts to develop more effective partnerships with each and every family though collaboration to resolve issues and concerns are addressing the awareness as well as the resources available to end disparities and inequities.

A number of other initiatives and trends are also apparent. In 2007, a national organization was formed through the Center of Applied Linguistics in Washington, D.C., to set a national dual-language research agenda. Support for current and future research that makes direct links for practitioners about dual-language learning can also contribute to improved quality to address issues of cultural, socioeconomic, linguistic, and ability diversity. Attention to articulation of professional standards and position statements from key organizations in early childhood (e.g., NAEYC; DEC; Zero to Three) that address issues of access and equity can also positively impact the improvements in practice that involves family relationships as central to young children's education and development.

The projects mentioned above are but a handful of examples of increasing efforts to examine and attend to continued challenges impacting equity in education, including those issues that impact children and families from socioeconomic, cultural, linguistic, and ability-diverse backgrounds in early care and education.

EMERGING TRENDS AND PROMISING PRACTICES

Enhancing the Knowledge Base

Research efforts increasingly provide evidence that support promising practices that will improve early intervention for all children with disabilities, including those who are culturally and linguistically diverse. These efforts may be in jeopardy in the near future given state and national fiscal funding constraints.

Longitudinal investigations of bilingual models of early childhood instruction, including dual-language programs, transition programs, and supplemental language supports, can, if funded, shed light on effectiveness of educational options and strategies that promote learning. Positive evidence of improved outcomes for all children when instructional strategies are embedded in a multitiered framework is emerging, especially when based upon the concept of a community of learners that includes parents as active participants in their children's early development and education. If support continues, the current focus on high-quality foundational/universal practices, such as use of research-based curriculums, universal screening, and progress monitoring, will provide accountability across the early childhood profession.

The funded research and demonstration projects that seek to understand how parent-professional partnerships can best be formed and sustained over time will offer insights for systemic changes at all levels of interaction. Emerging research sets the trend for improvement in practices that include all children regardless of ability, languages spoken, and cultures of origin, through engagement of parents as partners in this effort. Research can also address issues of personnel preparation focused on teacher quality, including ongoing investigations of effectiveness of family-centered, culturally competent, and culturally responsive practices. Continued funding of projects and research geared towards promising solutions to persistent dilemmas of social justice and equity is also needed. Research and its funding are issues that need to be addressed if we are to achieve desired outcomes that increase our knowledge base when partnering with families to improve educational practices that impact our youngest learners with disabilities.

Parent Education and Supports

Another promising practice involves sustained focus on parent engagement through parent education and support. Active engagement of families in early intervention has proven a viable model, fostering children's growth and development during the critical early childhood years. Many parents are eager to learn more about how they can foster their children's growth and development at home and what options are available and developmentally appropriate for early childhood education and intervention. At another level, the focus on prevention and early identification of challenges inherent in multitiered frameworks for instruction, currently being implemented in early care and education settings, holds promise of fostering active engagement of each and every child's family in their child's education. Prevention programs can lead to systemic changes that promote early identification, early intervention, and equity of access to high-quality early education educational opportunities. Projects like the nationally funded parent information and resource centers that foster and support parent-to-parent networking have proven effective in actively engaging parents and family members in learning about options for educational programs, their rights and responsibilities related to education of their children, and advocacy for their children with disabilities through development of strong parent-school partnerships. Parent leadership programs and opportunities at all levels in early childhood education can feed the desired outcomes of active parent participation predictive of positive outcomes for all children.

Adoption of Family-Centered, Culturally Competent, and Responsive Practices

Given current demographic trends reviewed in this chapter, there is no question that adoption of family-centered, culturally competent, and responsive practices is a current trend and a focus for improvement. Early interventionists that recognize the uniqueness of each and every family are central to success in promoting children's development and learning. Strategies and programs that enhance relationships with families based upon mutual respect, reciprocity, and communication through anchored understanding are considered essential to building partnerships with families that can effect change. Widespread adoption of family-centered and culturally competent attitudes, knowledge, and skills by early intervention professionals is a promising practice that hopefully will continue to drive needed change in our early intervention and education systems.

KEY MESSAGES

This chapter has described issues associated with the changing population receiving early intervention services now and in the future. It explores implications for professionals working with their families. Specific strategies and evidence-based practices that can improve relationships with families and directly impact the learning of young children with disabilities during the early childhood years are described. Family voices, stories, and perspectives are woven throughout with research citations to clarify as well as document the relevance of information shared. Reiteration of a key message that each and every child and family is deserving of *individual consideration*, regardless of their cultural, linguistic, or socioeconomic backgrounds, or differing abilities and identified challenges, pervades discussions. Information that enhances our understanding of culture and its relationship to language is considered integral to an understanding of how to build relationships and partnerships with families who represent diverse cultures.

REFERENCES

Abedi, J. (2006). The No Child Left Behind Act and English language learners: Assessment and accountability issues. *Educational Researcher, 33*, 4–14.

Anderson, P. P., & Fenichel, E. S. (1989). *Serving culturally diverse families of infants and toddlers with disabilities*. Rockville, MD: National Center for Clinical Infant Programs. Retrieved from http://eric.ed.gov/PDFS/ED318174.pdf

Artiles, A. J., & Trent, S. C. (1994). Overrepresentation of minority students in special education: A continued debate. *Journal of Special Education, 22*, 410–436.

August, D., & Hakuta, K. (1997). *Improving Schooling for Language-Minority Children*. Washington, DC: National Academy Press.

Barrera, I., & Corso, R. (2003). *Skilled dialogue: Strategies for responding to cultural diversity*. Baltimore: Paul H. Brookes.

Bialystok, E. (2001). Bilingualism in development: Language, literacy, and cognition. New York: Cambridge University Press.

Boylan, E., & White, S. (2010). Formula for success: Adding high-quality pre-k to state school funding formulas. Washington, DC: PEW Center on the States. Retrieved from http://www.pewcenteronthestates.org/uploadedFiles/Formula_for_Success.pdf?n=913

Bruns, D. A., & Corso, R. (2001). Working with culturally and linguistically diverse families. Retrieved from ERIC Digest, http://www.ericdigests.org/2002-2/diverse.htm

Burns, M. K., Appleton, J. J., & Stehouwer, J. D. (2005). Meta-analytic review of responsiveness-to-intervention research: Examining field-based and research-implemented models. Journal of Psychoeducational Assessment, 23, 381–394.

Buysse, V., Castro, D., & Peisner-Feinberg, E. (2010). Effects of personnel development program on classroom practices and outcomes for Latino dual language learners. *Early Childhood Research Quarterly, 25*(2), 194–206.

Capps, R., Michael, F., Ost, J., Reardon-Anderson, J., & Passel, J. (2004). *The health and well-being of young children of immigrants*. Washington, DC: Urban Institute.

Castro, D., Peisner-Feinberg, E., Buysse, V., & Gillanders, C. (2010). Language and literacy development of Latino dual language learners: Promising instructional practices. In O. N. Saracho & B. Spodek (Ed.), *Contemporary Perspectives in Early Childhood Education Series*. Charlotte, NC: Information Age Publishing.

Chen, D., Brekken, L., & Chan, S. (1998). *Project Craft: Culturally responsive and family focused training*. Van Nuys, CA: Child Development media.

Child Learning Center (CLC). (1999). *Pathways: A child and family journey*. Boulder, CO: Department of Speech, Language, and Hearing Science, University of Colorado.

Coleman, M. R., Buysse, V., & Neitzel, J. (2006). *Recognition and response: An early intervening system for young children at-risk for learning disabilities. Full report*. Chapel Hill: University of North Carolina, FPG Child Development Institute.

Coleman, R., Roth, F., & West, T. (2009). *Roadmap to Pre-K RTI: Applying response to intervention in preschool settings*, New York: National Center for Learning Disabilities. Available at http://www.florida-rti.org/Resources/_docs/roadmaptoprekrti.pdf

De Valenzuela, J. S., Copeland, S. R., Huaqing Qi, C., & Park, M. (2006). Examining educational equity: Revisiting the disproportionate representation of minority students in special education. *Exceptional Children, 72*, 425–441.

Dinnebeil, L. A., & Rule, S. (1994). Variables that influence collaboration between parents and service coordinators. *Journal of Early Intervention, 18*(4), 361–379.

Dunst, C., Trivette, C., & Hamby, D. W. (2008). *Research synthesis and meta-analysis of studies of family centered practice*. Asheville, NC: Winterberry Press.

Espinosa, L. (2008). Challenging common myths about young English language learners. *Foundation for Child Development, 8*, 2–11.

Fadiman, A. (1997). *The spirit catches you and you fall down*: New York: Farrar, Straus & Giroux.

Forum on Child and Family Statistics. (2010). *America's children in brief: Key national indicators of well-being*, Retrieved from http://www.childstats.gov

Genesee, F. (2008). Early dual language learning. *Zero to Three, 9*, 17–23.

Genesee, F., Paradis, J., & Crago, M. (2004). *Dual Language Development and Disorders*. Baltimore: Paul H. Brookes.

Goldstein, B. (2004). *Bilingual Language Development and Disorders*. Baltimore: Paul H. Brookes.

Guiberson, M. (2009). Hispanic representation in special education: Patterns and implications. *Preventing School Failure, 53*(3), 167–175.

Hakuta, K. (1986). *Mirror of language: The debate on bilingualism*. New York: Basic Books.

Hall, E. (1976). *Beyond Culture*. New York: Anchor Books.

Hardin, B. J., Mereoiu, M., Hung, H., & Roach-Scott, M. (2009). Investigating parent and professional perspectives concerning special education services for preschool Latino children. *Early Childhood Education Journal, 37*, 93–102.

Harry, B., Kalyanpur, M., & Day, M. (1999). *Building cultural reciprocity with families: Case studies in special education*. Baltimore: Paul H. Brookes.

Hepburn, K. S. (2004) *Building culturally and linguistically competent services to support young children, families and their school readiness*. Baltimore: Annie E. Casey Foundation.

Hernandez, D. J. (2004). Demographic change and the life circumstances of immigrant families. *The Future of Children, 14*(2) (Special issue, Children of Immigrant Families), 17–48.

House Memorial 5 Task Force on Young Children and Families. (1990). *First steps to a community-based coordinated continuum of care for New Mexico children and families*. (Available from Polly Arango, P.O. Box 338, Algodones, NM, 87001).

Kayser, H. (Ed.) (2008). *Educating Latino preschool children*. San Diego, CA: Plural.

Keller-Allen, C. (2006). *English language learners with disabilities: Identification and other state policies and issues*. Alexandria, VA: National Association of State Directors of Special Education. Retrieved from http://www.projectforum.org/docs/EnglishLanguageLearnerswithDisabilities-IdentificationandOtherStatePoliciesandIssues.pdf

Kipp, D. (2007). *Keeping a language alive*. Missoula, MT: The Missoulian.

Kohnert, K. (2008). *Language disorders in bilingual children and adults*, San Diego, CA: Plural.

Kohnert, K., Yim, D., Nett, K., Kan, P. F., Duran, L. (2005). Intervention with linguistically diverse preschool children: A focus on development of home language. *Language, Speech and Hearing Service in the Schools, 26*, 251–263.

Krashen, S. (1999). *Condemned without a trial: Bogus arguments against bilingual education*. Portsmouth, NH: Heinemann.

Lindholm-Leary, K. J. (2005). The rich promise of two-way immersion. *Educational Leadership, 62*, 56–59.

Lindholm-Leary, K., & Borsato, B. (2006). Academic achievement. In F. Genesee, K. Lindholm-Leary, W. Saunders, & D. Christian (Eds.), *Educating English language learners: A synthesis of research evidence* (pp. 176–222). New York: Cambridge University Press.

Lynch, E. W., & Hanson, M. J. (Eds.). (2004). *Developing crosscultural competence: A guide for working with children and their families* (3rd ed.). Baltimore: Paul H. Brookes.

Maude, S., Catlett, C., Moore, S., Sánchez, S., & Thorp E. (2006). Educating and training students to work with culturally, linguistically, and ability-diverse young children and their families. *Zero to Three, 2*(3), 28–35.

Moore, S. M., Eiserman, W., Pérez-Méndez, C., & Beatty, J. (1998). The Spectrum Project, UCB: Boulder.

Moore, S. M., & Pérez-Méndez, C. (2003). *Cultural contexts for early intervention.* Rockville, MD: American Speech-Language-Hearing Association.

Moore, S. M., & Pérez-Méndez, C. (2005a). *Beyond words: Effective use of cultural mediators, interpreters and translators,* Boulder CO: Landlocked Films. (Available from http://www.landlockedfilms.com)

Moore, S., & Pérez-Méndez, C. (2005b). Parent and family involvement: Module 6. In *English language learners with exceptional needs.* Golden, CO: Meta Associates.

Moore, S. M., & Pérez-Méndez, C. (2005c). *The Story about El Grupo: A parent education and support group.* Boulder, Co: Landlocked Films. (Available from http://www.landlockedfilms.com)

Moore, S. M., & Pérez-Méndez, C. (2006). Working with linguistically diverse families in early Intervention: Misconceptions and Missed Opportunities, *Seminars in Speech and Language, 27,* 187–198.

Moore, S. M., Pérez-Méndez, C., & Boerger, K. (2006). Meeting the needs of culturally and linguistically diverse families in early language and literacy intervention. In L. Justice (Ed.), *Clinical Approaches to Emergent Literacy Intervention.* San Diego, CA: Plural.

NAEYC. (1995). *Responding to linguistic and cultural diversity recommendations for effective early childhood education: A position statement.* Washington, DC: Author.

Nieto, S. (2000). *The light in their eyes: Creating multicultural learning communities.* New York: Teachers College Press.

Ortiz, A. A., & Yates, J. R. (1983). Incidence of exceptionality among Hispanics: Implications for manpower planning. *NABE Journal of Research and Practice, 7,* 41–54.

Passel, J. & Cohn, D'V. (2008). *U.S. population projections: 2005–2050.* Washington, DC: PEW Research Center.

Pérez-Méndez, C., & Moore, S. M. (2004). *Culture and language: Respecting family choice.* Boulder, CO: Landlocked Films. (Available from http://www.landlockedfilms.com)

Restrepo, M. A., Castilla, A., Schwanenflugel, S., Neuharth-Pritchett, P., Hamilton, C., & Arboleda, A. (2010). Effects of a supplemental Spanish oral language program on sentence length, complexity, and grammaticality in Spanish-speaking children attending English-only preschools, *Language, Speech, and Hearing Services in Schools, 41,* 3–13.

Sánchez, S. (1999a). Learning from the stories of culturally and linguistically diverse families and communities. *Remedial and Special Education, 20,* 351–359.

Sánchez, S. Y. (1999b). Issues of language and culture impacting the early care of young Latino children. *Child Care Bulletin, 24.* Retrieved from http://nccic.org/ccb/issue24.html

Sánchez, S., & Thorp, E. (2008). Teaching to transform: Infusing cultural and linguistic diversity. In P. Winton, J. McCollum, & C. Catlett (Eds.), *Practical approaches to early childhood professional development: Evidence, strategies, and resources* (pp. 81–97). Washington, DC: Zero to Three Press.

Santos, R. M., Corso, R. M., & Fowler, S. A. (2005). *Working with linguistically diverse families.* Champaign, IL: CLAS.

Sue, D. W., Ivey, A. E. & Pederson, P. B. (1996). *A theory of multicultural counseling and therapy.* Florence, KY: Brookes Cole Publishers.

Tabors, P. O. (2008). *One child: Two languages* (2nd ed.). Baltimore: Paul H. Brookes.

Tatum, B. D. (2003). *"Why are all the Black kids sitting together in the cafeteria?" and other conversations about race.* New York: Basic Books.

Thorp, E. (1997). Increasing opportunities for partnership with culturally and linguistically diverse families. *Intervention in School and Clinic, 32,* 261–269.

Van Kleeck, A. (1994). Potential cultural bias in training parents as conversational partners with their children who have delays in language development. *American Journal of Speech-Language Pathology, 1,* 67–78.

Westby, C. (1990). Ethnographic interviewing: Asking the right questions to the right people in the right ways. *Journal of Childhood Communication Disorders, 13* (1), 101–111.

Westby, C. (2009). Considerations when working successfully with culturally and linguistically diverse families in assessment and intervention of communication disorders, *Seminars in Speech and language,* 30(4) 279–289.

Winsler, A., Diaz, R. M., Espinosa, L., & Rodriguez, J. L. (1999). When learning a second language does not mean losing the first: Bilingual language development in low-income, Spanish-speaking children attending bilingual preschool. *Child Development, 70,* 349–362.

Winton, P., McCollum, J. A., & Catlett, C. (2008). *Practical approaches to early childhood professional development: Evidence, strategies, and resources.* Washington, DC: Zero to Three Press.

Wong Fillmore, L. (1991). When learning one language means losing the first. *Early Childhood Research Quarterly,* 6(3), 323–346.

Yoshida, H. (2008). The cognitive consequences of early bilingualism. *Journal of Zero to Three, 29,* 26–30.

Chapter 2

Recognition and Response: Response to Intervention for Prekindergarten

Ellen Peisner-Feinberg, Virginia Buysse,
LeeMarie A. Benshoff, and Elena P. Soukaku

KEY CONTEXTS FOR TIERED MODELS IN EARLY CHILDHOOD

S everal trends in the United States have focused national attention on early education and helped to influence new directions in this regard: the emphasis on high-quality programs and services; the school readiness movement; and the importance of early detection, prevention, and intervention for learning difficulties.

HIGH-QUALITY PROGRAMS

The quality of early care and education has been at the forefront of research in the early childhood field for several decades. There is now sufficient empirical evidence to show that the quality of early childhood programs is an important determinant of children's social, language, and cognitive outcomes, as well as their school readiness skills (National Institute of Child Health and Human Development Early Child Care Research Network [NICHD ECCRN], 2000, 2002, 2003; Peisner-Feinberg & Burchinal, 1997; Peisner-Feinberg et al., 2001; Vandell, 2004). As a part of a high-quality program, early childhood teachers are expected to implement a curriculum that aligns with program and early learning standards and to make sound instructional decisions for each and every child (Copple & Bredekamp, 2009; National Association for the Education of Young Children [NAEYC] & National Association of Early Childhood Specialists in

State Departments of Education [NAECS/SDE], 2009). Recently, definitions of program quality have expanded to incorporate ways in which teachers can customize teaching and learning to address the needs of an increasingly diverse population of young children and families. Tiered models of instruction described later in this chapter help teachers recognize which children require additional instructional supports to learn key skills and provide teachers with specific interventions that are matched to these children's learning needs.

SCHOOL READINESS

There is now widespread consensus that experiences during the first five years of life provide the foundation for children's development in language, reasoning, problem solving, social skills, behavior, and adjustment to school. The nature of these early experiences affects children's later school success as well as their continued learning and development (Belsky et al., 2007; National Research Council & Institute of Medicine, 2003). Specific skills in the areas of language, literacy, and mathematics now are included in the definition of school readiness for children enrolled in prekindergarten programs and reflected in federal and state program standards that guide early education practices. The growing emphasis on children's academic learning during prekindergarten has been accompanied by the need for teachers to monitor children's progress in learning in these areas, to determine when children are experiencing difficulties in learning, and to use this information to inform decisions and select evidence-based intervention approaches that are beneficial in supporting children's learning needs.

EARLY INTERVENING

For children birth to 3 years old with developmental delays or identified disabilities, the Individuals with Disabilities Education Act (IDEA) provides a comprehensive system of early intervention services and appropriate public education and related services for children with disabilities. Tiered models such as those described in this chapter extend instructional supports to children who may not be eligible for early intervention or special education services, but who show signs of needing additional help from teachers to learn—a concept called *early intervening* because the focus is on helping children before they are referred to special education. Early intervening provided within the context of the general education curriculum can be used to provide additional supports for children at risk for school failure and to extend and complement existing special education services for young children with disabilities.

ORIGINS OF RECOGNITION AND RESPONSE

RtI for School-Age Children

The R&R model for prekindergarten children has its origins in Response to Intervention (RtI) models designed for use with school-age children. Regardless of the grade level or type of classroom, teachers need to provide instruction for children with a range of ability levels. For example, while one elementary school student may struggle with trying to read short words, another student may be reading chapter books with ease. With limited hours in the school day and many different children to teach, teachers need a system to help them best serve *all* students. Prior to the introduction of RtI, most schools used a discrepancy model to determine which students had learning disabilities. In the discrepancy model, schools would wait until children were failing to determine whether they qualified for additional educational services and supports. Typically, teachers would refer students who were performing well below the expected level for their age and/or grade for formal evaluations. From there, school psychologists would administer standardized tests to measure students' cognitive functioning (i.e., IQ) and academic skills. If a "significant" discrepancy was found between a student's cognitive and academic test scores, indicating that cognitive ability was higher than academic performance, that individual would be eligible to receive special education services. One of the chief problems with the discrepancy model is that some students may not meet the required discrepancy upon their first evaluation and will continue to struggle in school. Some of these students may meet eligibility requirements for special education services later in their schooling, but at the cost of months or even years of experiencing academic difficulties.

RtI is a system that was developed as an alternative approach to the discrepancy model. RtI focuses on intervening early to address learning difficulties as soon as problems appear, rather than waiting for children to experience school failure. There are numerous approaches to implementing RtI with school-age children (see Fuchs, 2003; Fuchs & Fuchs, 2002; Fuchs, Fuchs, & Compton, 2004; Haager, Klinger, & Vaughn, 2007; Jimerson, Burns, & VanDerHeyden, 2007; Marston, Muyskens, Lau, & Canter, 2003; Speece, Case, & Molloy, 2003; Torgesen et al., 1999; Vaughn & Fuchs, 2003; Vaughn, Linan-Thompson, & Hickman, 2003; Vellutino et al., 1996). However, RtI is generally based on three common components: (1) the use of a research-based core curriculum and effective instruction for all students, (2) a data-based decision-making system in which teachers gather information (i.e., data) to assess students' skills to determine who needs additional help and what types of supports for learning should be provided, and (3) planned instructional methods for helping students who need additional assistance in the classroom (i.e., interventions). RtI integrates these key components through a tiered model of instruction. Tiered models offer an approach in which teaching methods and interventions become increasingly intensive at each tier (or level) of the model, as needed by children.

Thus far, RtI has been utilized primarily with school-age children. It is currently considered an emerging practice within the fields of early childhood education and early intervention for children birth to age 5. Recognition & Response (R&R), the focus of the present chapter, is a model of RtI specifically adapted for use with prekindergarten children ages 3 to 5 years old.

Evidence for the Effectiveness of RtI

RtI has become a topic of increasing interest over the past several years, with some research studies demonstrating its success in the classroom. Research findings have indicated that RtI is particularly effective when implemented in the early grades and has resulted both in positive outcomes for children's learning and reductions in the use of special education services by schools using this approach. Given the widespread interest in this topic, user-friendly practice guides recently have been developed by the U.S. Department of Education to summarize the currently available evidence and offer recommendations to educators for implementing RtI.

A meta-analysis of 24 studies involving school-age children offers evidence of the effects of RtI at both the child and the school level (Burns, Appleton, & Stehouwer, 2005). This meta-analysis concluded that students attending schools implementing RtI demonstrated greater growth in academic skills, more time on task, and better task completion compared to those attending schools not implementing RtI. The schools implementing RtI also had fewer referrals to special education, fewer students placed in special education, and fewer students retained in a grade (i.e., not promoted to the subsequent grade) compared to other schools. Additionally, fewer students attending schools that implemented RtI were identified as having a learning disability compared to other schools; this finding countered the concern that the use of RtI may result in larger numbers of children being identified as having a learning disability.

Two practice guides by the Institute of Education Sciences (IES), one addressing the use of RtI to improve reading skills in primary grades and the other related to math skills in elementary and middle school, were developed based on the findings of a panel of experts including both researchers and practitioners (Gersten et al., 2008; Gersten et al., 2009). These guides summarize the evidence for the effectiveness of the key components of RtI, as well as indicate the need for further research. Regarding the first component of RtI, an effective core curriculum for all students, the guides note that there is limited research evidence available to inform decisions about the most effective curricula to use for teaching both reading and math in the elementary grades. They emphasize the importance of the second key component of RtI, assessment, as critical for ensuring that children who need additional instructional supports in reading or math are appropriately identified. Assessment within an RtI framework is discussed in the context of conducting universal screenings of children's reading and math skills and monitoring the progress of children who are determined to be at risk for difficulties. The guides state that there is empirical support showing that universal screening measures can predict children's future performance in these areas, and that progress monitoring can help increase teachers' awareness of students' skills, resulting in a positive effect on the instructional decisions that teachers make. Students who demonstrate insufficient progress, based on assessment data, should receive more intensive instruction. Regarding the third key component of RtI, intervention, the guides indicate strong evidence of the effectiveness of targeted interventions in both reading and math for elementary school students who were identified as at risk for later difficulties in these areas. The guides stress that these targeted interventions should be explicit and systematic, and should address foundational skills in each academic area (such as focusing on letter sounds for kindergarten children needing additional help with learning to read).

A separate research synthesis conducted on studies evaluating the efficacy of RtI among younger elementary school students found that when RtI was implemented in kindergarten, fewer children were referred for special education services later in their schooling (Coleman, Buysse, & Neitzel, 2006). This finding suggests that implementing RtI as early as kindergarten, and perhaps even earlier in prekindergarten as in the R&R model, may increase children's experiences of academic success, particularly for those who may be at risk for learning difficulties.

Although there is some evidence to support the efficacy of RtI, nearly all the research has been conducted with school-age children. In the field of early childhood education, current literature relating to the use of RtI in prekindergarten settings remains largely theoretical. Despite this lack of research, there is growing support for the use of RtI in early childhood, as it is consistent with the priorities for educational practice. Commonalities between the goals of RtI and of general early childhood educational practices include a focus on providing high-quality education and care to all children, an emphasis on the importance of educating children in natural and inclusive settings, and the provision of interventions matched to children's needs (Fox, Carta, Strain, Dunlap, & Hemmeter, 2010).

Only a few tiered instructional approaches modeled after RtI exist in early childhood. A review of the various tiered intervention models designed for children up to age 5 concluded that these models generally were congruent with RtI, as they all promoted high-quality learning environments, practices, and interventions to meet children's needs (VanDerHeyden & Snyder, 2006). In contrast to the RtI models for older children, the models for younger children tend to focus on naturalistic interventions to support social-emotional and behavioral functioning rather than interventions to promote academic skills such as reading and math. One key component of RtI that was noticeably absent from most models for younger children, however, was the use of assessment information about children's skills to plan and evaluate instruction (i.e., data-based decision making).

Table 2.1 summarizes the three primary tiered models currently available for early childhood settings that utilize at least some key elements of RtI. R&R can be distinguished from the other tiered models because it specifically addresses academic learning for young children (e.g., language, literacy, math) and includes *all* of the key components of RtI (a core curriculum and intentional teaching for all children; gathering information about children's skills; increasingly intensive, research-based interventions; and a collaborative problem-solving

Table 2.1 Tiered Models Currently Available for Use in Early Childhood

Model	Description	Target Population
Recognition & Response (Recognition & Response Implementation Guide, 2008)	A system that links assessment, instruction, and targeted interventions to support children's learning and development in multiple domains (e.g., literacy, language, math)	Children with learning difficulties/disabilities
Building Blocks (Sandall & Schwartz, 2008)	Instructional strategies organized by level of intensity to support participation, engagement, and learning in inclusive settings	Children with disabilities
Teaching Pyramid (Hemmeter, Ostrosky, & Fox, 2006)	Instructional strategies organized by level of intensity to support children's social-emotional development and help teachers address children's challenging behaviors	Children with social-emotional difficulties

process to support instructional decision making). R&R offers the most comprehensive system designed for use in early childhood education that is aligned with the principles of RtI.

The first study of the implementation of R&R in prekindergarten classrooms focused on the area of language and literacy skills (Buysse & Peisner-Feinberg, 2009). The study found that while children who received the targeted intervention in language and literacy scored lower than their classmates (as would be expected), they made greater pre- to post-intervention gains in scores on measures of letter naming, vocabulary, sound awareness, and print knowledge. Moreover, teachers who participated in the study reported that the model was highly useful and easy to implement.

KEY COMPONENTS OF R&R

The R&R model can be understood as a system for responding more efficiently to children's learning needs by linking assessment information that teachers gather on children's skills with everyday classroom instruction. The focus of R&R is on helping early childhood teachers organize and implement their instructional practices more systematically to better meet the educational needs of all children. The R&R framework guides teachers to make informed, data-based decisions regarding the level of instructional intensity children need across various content areas (e.g., emergent literacy, language, and math).

The R&R system consists of three key components: recognition, response, and collaborative problem solving. *Recognition* in R&R involves gathering assessment information on children's development, including universal screening of all children and progress monitoring for some children who may need additional instructional supports to learn. *Response* in R&R relates to the instruction that teachers plan and offer to children. Elements of the response component include general instruction through the provision of a high-quality core curriculum and intentional teaching for all children and targeted interventions for some students who show signs of learning difficulties in areas such as language and literacy or math. Recognizing and responding to children's needs effectively and efficiently is facilitated through a *collaborative problem-solving* process, the third component of R&R. Through collaborative problem solving, teachers, specialists, and other professionals work together to link information about children's skills and progress with the kinds and levels of instructional methods that can best support their learning needs.

Each of the R&R components is provided in the context of a tiered approach in which each child receives the level of instructional support needed to learn. The R&R system is designed to provide high-quality instruction for *all* children, along with targeted interventions for *some* children and more intensive instructional strategies for a *few* children. Figure 2.1 shows the key components of this tiered model, and Table 2.2 presents an overview of how each component is implemented across the three tiers.

Recognition: Universal Screening and Progress Monitoring

In the R&R model, the recognition component consists of the systematic use of assessment data gathered through universal screening and progress monitoring. The first element, universal screening, involves gathering assessment information on skill levels for all children in a prekindergarten program to determine whether individual children might require additional help to master certain skills. For example, a

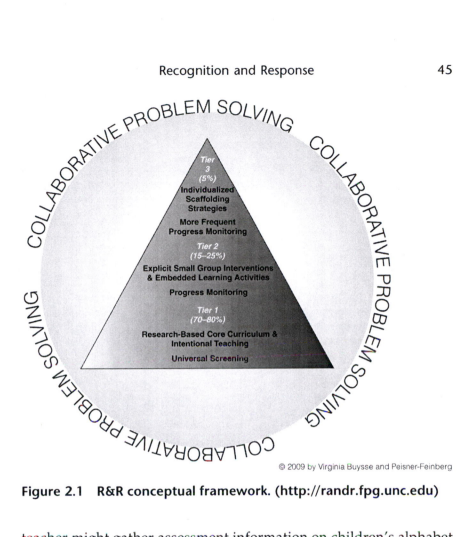

Figure 2.1   R&R conceptual framework. (http://randr.fpg.unc.edu)

teacher might gather assessment information on children's alphabet knowledge or counting skills. Teachers then use this screening information to recognize which children might need additional interventions.

Universal screening generally occurs three times a year, on a fall, winter, and spring schedule. Based on these assessment results, if most children meet key learning benchmarks, it can be assumed that the general instruction is of sufficient quality. However, the universal screening data may still indicate that there are some children who are not making adequate progress, even with a good core curriculum and other intentional teaching activities.

The second element of the recognition component of R&R, progress monitoring, is a systematic process for teachers to further measure the progress of those children who are receiving targeted interventions (as determined by the universal screening results). Teachers monitor progress by periodically assessing children's skills during the

Table 2.2   Implementation of Recognition and Response: Tiers 1, 2, and 3

Tier/Focus	Recognition	Response	Collaborative Problem Solving
Tier 1: *All* children	Universal screening	Research-based core curriculum and intentional teaching	Interpret screening results and develop intervention plans
Tier 2 *Some* children	Progress monitoring	Explicit small-group interventions and embedded learning opportunities	Interpret progress monitoring results and adjust intervention plans
Tier 3 *A few* children	Additional progress monitoring	Continued use of explicit and embedded interventions, with added individualized scaffolding	Interpret progress monitoring results and adjust intervention plans

intervention period to see how well individual children are responding to these added instructional interventions. There may still be a few students who do not reach their goals based on progress-monitoring data and therefore need an even more intensive level of instructional support. For these children, teachers may include additional assessments to monitor their progress and make adjustments to the interventions as needed.

To gather information on children, teachers ideally select tools that can be used both for universal screening with all children during the year as well as for monitoring the progress of some children receiving additional learning supports. Such tools share a number of important characteristics. They measure both children's level and rate of growth; that is, how well a child performs at a given point in time and how much a child learns over time. Also, these tools are not tied to a specific curriculum; rather, they measure children's skills within key domains of learning (e.g., language and literacy skills, math skills). In this way, teachers can use the results from their assessments to make decisions about the particular curricula and interventions that best meet children's learning needs. Furthermore, universal screening and progress-monitoring measures are designed to be used multiple times throughout the school year. As such, these measures need to be quick and easy for teachers to administer, generally around 5–10 minutes per assessment.

Response: Instruction and Intervention

The response component in the R&R model refers to the core instruction offered to all children as well as the more targeted interventions that are provided for some children who require additional help to learn. In R&R, classroom instruction and interventions are implemented through a tiered approach; that is, they are organized hierarchically from least intensive to most intensive to reflect how directive and involved a teacher is according to children's learning needs.

According to this approach, Tier 1, the first level of instruction in the R&R model, involves providing a high-quality, effective core curriculum along with intentional teaching of key school readiness skills for all children in the classroom. A high-quality, effective curriculum is one that is based on research evidence; is developmentally appropriate for the children's ages; and is comprehensive, covering all domains of learning. A second aspect of instruction for all children at Tier 1 is intentional teaching of critical skills for school readiness within the key domains of learning (i.e., language, literacy, math), such as vocabulary, story concepts, or simple number skills. Intentional teaching entails thoughtfully and planfully implementing specific aspects of the curriculum and instructional approaches to ensure that children are given regular opportunities to develop critical skills and achieve learning goals. Intentional teaching occurs through the purposeful organization of the classroom environment and provision of planned, developmentally appropriate activities to offer opportunities for children to learn and develop these important skills. A high-quality core curriculum along with intentional teaching of key skills should enable most children to make adequate progress in learning at Tier 1.

At Tier 2, the second level of instruction in the R&R model, teachers make specific adjustments to their instruction for children who require additional supports to learn based on the results of the universal screening data. To enhance learning, teachers implement targeted interventions with small groups of children (generally 3–6 children) who have similar learning goals. In R&R, the interventions at Tier 2 take place in addition to the general curriculum and classroom routines. Children receiving these targeted interventions still fully participate in the instructional activities offered at Tier 1.

The Tier 2 interventions are designed to address specific skills in key academic areas such as language, literacy, and math. The targeted interventions are based on domain-specific curricula, with research evidence to support their effectiveness. Such interventions provide teachers with a sequenced set of instructional activities or lessons to explicitly teach specific skills. They are designed to be used in small groups (generally 3–5 children) and address skills that are developmentally appropriate for the selected age group. For example, a teacher might form a small group of children to implement a research-based intervention for language and literacy development, which teaches skills such as vocabulary, sound awareness, and letter recognition. These small-group lessons would take place for approximately 15 minutes a day while the rest of the class is engaged in other activities. In R&R, such Tier 2 interventions typically occur over an 8- to 10-week period.

The explicit small-group interventions at Tier 2 are complemented by embedded learning activities. These are designed to extend children's learning by offering additional opportunities to practice, generalize, and maintain skills outside the small-group intervention time, such as during center time or during other Tier 1 activities. Teachers create embedded learning activities by intentionally adapting or enriching existing contexts for teaching and learning within Tier 1, including the learning environment, activities, and routines. Examples of embedded learning activities include arranging the environment to support specific skills, such as adding signs and labels in the classroom to support the development of print concepts; or modifying aspects of the curriculum, such as adding a picture-naming game to centers to support the development of vocabulary skills.

At Tier 3, the response component consists of the addition of more intensive scaffolding strategies to further support children's learning within the Tier 2 interventions. These Tier 3 interventions are teaching strategies that have been found to be effective through research and are selected on an individual basis for a few children who require further support to learn certain skills. An example of a scaffolding strategy might include modeling or showing the child how to respond to a question during a storybook reading activity or having a peer help the child with a letter-naming game. These strategies are designed to further support the small-group interventions and embedded learning activities offered in Tier 2. Therefore, scaffolding strategies are provided in addition to the Tier 1 activities and the Tier 2 interventions to ensure that these children are receiving the level of instructional support needed.

Collaborative Problem Solving

Within R&R, collaborative problem solving offers a process by which teachers, parents, and specialists can work together to plan various

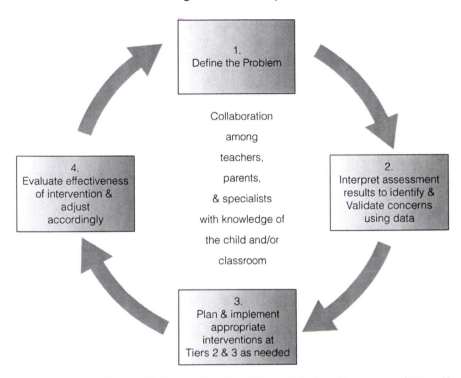

Figure 2.2   The Collaborative Problem Solving Process. (http://randr.fpg.unc.edu)

levels of instructional supports and assess how well children respond to them. Collaborative problem solving has its origins in a framework first described by Bergan and his colleagues (Bergan, 1977; Bergan & Kratochwill, 1990). The R&R model incorporates a process of collaborative problem solving, as depicted in Figure 2.2.

In the R&R model, programs establish core problem-solving teams to make decisions based on this framework. The starting point in this process is to define the problem by reviewing assessment information on children. Next, the collaborative problem-solving team works together to analyze assessment results to make data-based decisions about needed adjustments in instruction. The next step in this process involves developing and implementing a plan for modifying instruction for some children based on the tiered instructional approach of the R&R model. Finally, the team needs to evaluate these modifications, including implementing a plan for monitoring children's progress and continuing to make needed instructional adjustments based on data. The problem-solving team also determines the times and ways for documenting and sharing information with others, including parents, professionals, and specialists.

FUTURE DIRECTIONS

R&R is an emerging practice in early childhood based closely on principles of RtI, but adapted for younger children enrolled in early care and education programs. The practices recommended within R&R are consistent with the current emphasis in early childhood education on high-quality curriculum and teaching, the importance of intervening early using research-based approaches, and the need to connect teaching and learning to positive outcomes for children and families. Although R&R holds promise for supporting learners in prekindergarten, additional research is needed with larger samples and across various content areas to provide further evidence of the model's effectiveness.

The early childhood field also needs policies, guidelines, and resources to support the implementation of R&R in prekindergarten at a broader level. Provisions within IDEA address the use of RtI for school-age children, with a particular emphasis on children in kindergarten through third grade. However, there are no specific provisions within IDEA or any other federal legislation that address R&R/RtI for young children in prekindergarten, child care, early intervention, or Head Start programs. The use of R&R in early childhood settings is intended to complement, not replace, existing special education services for children with disabilities. R&R can complement these special services by helping teachers organize their instructional supports for children with disabilities who have an Individualized Education Program (IEP). It is important that educators not use R&R to delay or deny services or referrals for children with identified disabilities or those for whom parents and teachers have serious concerns.

Because R&R is an emerging early childhood practice, all of the factors necessary to support its implementation in prekindergarten classrooms are not yet known. Some decisions will need to be made at the program level, and teachers will need the full support of administrators, specialists, and families to use R&R effectively in their classrooms. In the meantime, studies are underway to help determine the best ways to implement these practices in early childhood classrooms and to expand the research evidence about the effectiveness of such

tiered instructional approaches for supporting learning and development for all young children.

References

Belsky, J., Vandell, D. L., Burchinal, M., Clarke-Stewart, K. A., McCartney, K., Owen, M. T., & NICHD Early Child Care Research Network. (2007). Are there long-term effects of early child care? *Child Development, 78*(2), 681–701. doi:10.111/j.1467-8624.2007.01021x

Bergan, J. (1977). *Behavioral consultation*. Columbus, OH: Merrill.

Bergan, J., & Kratochwill, T. R. (1990). *Behavioral consultation and therapy.* New York: Plenum.

Burns, M. K., Appleton, J. J., & Stehouwer, J. D. (2005). Meta-analytic review of responsiveness-to-intervention research: Examining field-based and research-implemented models. *Journal of Psychoeducational Assessment, 23*(4), 381–394. doi:doi:10.1177/073428290502300406

Buysse, V., & Peisner-Feinberg, E. S. (2009). *Recognition and response: Findings from the first implementation study.* Retrieved from http://randr.fpg.unc.edu/presentations

Coleman, M. R., Buysse, V., & Neitzel, J. (2006). *Recognition and response: An early intervening system for young children at-risk for learning disabilities. Full report.* Chapel Hill: University of North Carolina, FPG Child Development Institute.

Copple, C., & Bredekamp, S. (Eds.) (2009). *Developmentally appropriate practice in early childhood programs serving children from birth through age 8* (3rd ed.). Washington, DC: NAEYC.

Fox, L., Carta, J., Strain, P. S., Dunlap, G., & Hemmeter, M. L. (2010). Response to intervention and the pyramid model. *Infants and Young Children, 23*(1), 3–13. doi:10.1097/IYC.06013e3181c816e2

Fuchs, D., Fuchs, L. S., & Compton, D. L. (2004). Identifying reading disabilities by responsiveness-to-instruction: Specifying measures and criteria. *Learning Disability Quarterly, 27*(4), 216–227.

Fuchs, L. S. (2003). Assessing intervention responsiveness: Conceptual and technical issues. *Learning Disabilities Research and Practice, 18*(3), 172–186. doi:10.111/1540-5826.00073

Fuchs, L., & Fuchs, D. (2002). Curriculum-based measurement: Describing competence, enhancing outcomes, evaluating treatment effects, and evaluating treatment nonresponders. *Peabody Journal of Education, 77*(2), 64–84.

Gersten, R., Beckmann, S., Clarke, B., Foegen, A., Marsh, L., Star, J. R., & Witzel, B. (2009). *Assisting students struggling with mathematics: Response to Intervention (RtI) for elementary and middle schools.* (NCEE 2009-4060). Washington, DC: National Center for Education Evaluation and Regional Assistance, Institute of Education Sciences, U.S. Department of Education. Retrieved from http://ies.ed.gov/ncee/wwc/publications/practiceguides

Gersten, R., Compton, D., Connor, C., Dimino, J., Santoro, L., Linan-Thompson, S., & Tilly, W. D. (2008). *Assisting students struggling with reading: Response to Intervention and multi-tier intervention for reading in the primary grades. A practice guide.* (NCEE

2009-4045).Washington, DC: National Center for Education Evaluation and Regional Assistance, Institute of Education Sciences, U.S. Department of Education. Retrieved from http://ies.ed.gov/ncee/wwc/publications/practiceguides

Haager, D., Klingner, J., & Vaughn, S. (2007). *Evidence-based reading practices for response to intervention*. Baltimore: Paul H. Brookes.

Hemmeter, M. L., Ostrosky, M., & Fox, L. (2006). Social and emotional foundations for early learning: A conceptual model for intervention. *School Psychology Review, 35*(4), 583–601.

Jimerson, S. R., Burns, M. K., & VanDerHeyden, A. M. (Eds.). (2007). *Handbook of response to intervention: The science and practice of assessment and intervention*. New York: Springer.

Marston, D., Muyskens, P., Lau, M., & Canter, A. (2003). Problem-solving model for decision making with high-incidence disabilities: The Minneapolis experience. *Learning Disabilities Research and Practice, 18*(3), 187–200. doi: 10.111/1540-5826.00074

National Association for the Education of Young Children and National Association of Early Childhood Specialists in State Departments of Education. (2009). *Where we stand on curriculum, assessment, and program evaluation*. Washington, DC: NAEYC.

National Research Council and Institute of Medicine. (2003). *Working families and growing kids: Caring for children and adolescents*. Committee on Family and Work Policies (E. Smolensky & J. A. Gootman, Eds.). Board on Children, Youth, and Families, Division of Behavioral and Social Sciences and Education. Washington, DC: National Academies Press.

National Institute of Child Health and Human Development (NICHD) Early Child Care Research Network. (2000). The relation of child care to cognitive and language development. *Child Development, 71*(4), 960–980. doi:10.111/1467-8624.00202

National Institute of Child Health and Human Development (NICHD) Early Child Care Research Network. (2002). Early child care and children's development prior to school entry: Results from the NICHD study of early child care. *American Educational Research Journal, 39*(1), 133–164.

National Institute of Child Health and Human Development (NICHD) Early Child Care Research Network. (2003). Does quality of child care affect child outcomes at age 4 1/2? *Developmental Psychology, 39*(3), 451–469.

Peisner-Feinberg, E. S., & Burchinal, M. R. (1997). Relations between preschool children's child-care experiences and concurrent development: The cost, quality, and outcomes study. *Merrill-Palmer Quarterly, 43*(3), 451–477.

Peisner-Feinberg, E. S., Burchinal, M. R., Clifford, R. M., Culkin, M. L., Howes, C., Kagan, S. L., & Yazejian, N. (2001). The relation of preschool child-care quality to children's cognitive and social developmental trajectories through second grade. *Child Development, 72*(5), 1534–1553. doi:10.1111/1467-8624.00364

Recognition and response implementation guide. (2008). Chapel Hill: University of North Carolina, FPG Child Development Institute.

Sandall, S. R., & Schwartz, I. S. (2008). *Building blocks for teaching preschoolers with special needs* (2nd ed.). Baltimore: Paul H. Brookes.

Speece, D. L., Case, L. P., & Molloy, D. E. (2003). Responsiveness to general education instruction as the first gate to learning disabilities identification. *Learning Disabilities Research and Practice, 18*(3), 147–156. doi:10.1111/1540-5826.00071

Torgesen, J. K., Wagner, R. K., Rashotte, C. A., Rose, E., Lindamood, P., Conway, T., & Garvan, C. (1999). Preventing reading failure in young children with phonological processing disabilities: Group and individual responses to instruction. *Journal of Educational Psychology, 91*(4), 579–593.

Vandell, D. L. (2004). Early child care: The known and the unknown. *Merrill-Palmer Quarterly, 50*(3), 387–414.

VanDerHeyden, A. M., & Snyder, P. (2006). Integrating frameworks from early childhood intervention and school psychology to accelerate growth for all young children. *School Psychology Review, 35*(4), 519–534.

Vaughn, S., & Fuchs, L. S. (2003). Redefining learning disabilities as inadequate response to instruction: The promise and potential problems. *Learning Disabilities Research and Practice, 18*(3), 137–146. doi:10.1111/1540-5826.00070

Vaughn, S., Linan-Thompson, S., & Hickman, P. (2003). Response to instruction as a means of identifying students with reading/learning disabilities. *Exceptional Children, 69*(4), 391–409.

Vellutino, F. R., Scanlon, D. M., Sipay, E. R., Small, S. G., Pratt, A., Chen, R., & Denckla, M. B. (1996). Cognitive profiles of difficult-to-remediate and readily remediated poor readers: Early intervention as a vehicle for distinguishing between cognitive and experiential deficits as basic causes of specific reading disability. *Journal of Educational Psychology, 88*(4), 601–638.

Chapter 3

Data-Driven Decision Making to Plan Programs and Promote Performance

Kristie Pretti-Frontczak, Stephen J. Bagnato,
Marisa Macy, and Dawn Burger Sexton

A ssessment in everyday environments is the key component to planning, monitoring, and evaluating effective early childhood intervention programs for young children with developmental delays and disabilities. Assessment is broadly defined "as a process of gathering information for the purpose of making decisions" (McLean, Wolery, & Bailey, 2004, p. 13). Interdisciplinary professionals in the fields of early intervention (EI) and early childhood special education (ECSE) use assessment to reach a series of critical decisions, and to take actions for the benefit of vulnerable children and families. Some of the critical decisions and actions may include:

- Confirming suspected delays in development
- Setting functional goals for intervention
- Designing individualized intervention strategies
- Modifying instruction and intervention based upon ongoing assessment
- Monitoring expected performance and progress
- Documenting parent and consumer satisfaction with services
- Evaluating the extent to which children are meeting state and federal benchmarks as a result of participation in the program

Despite the critical nature of these decisions and actions, EI/ECSE professionals confront challenges as they assess young children. First, agencies often develop policies and mandate practices that are impractical, invalid, and, arguably, unethical. For example, measures are required that do not have documented technical adequacy and/or validation for specific early intervention purposes. Often, the most popular measures require limited response modes that make it impossible for children with prominent functional limitations (i.e., vision, hearing, communication, motor, behavior) to demonstrate their underlying capabilities.

Second, personnel may lack the training and ongoing administrative support needed to use measures faithfully, and/or to interpret and apply assessment information to better serve young children and their families. Finally, EI/ECSE professionals find that policies and practices regarding assessment for early intervention are often frustrating and contrary to recommended professional standards.

In the chapter, we have three objectives to help interdisciplinary professionals conduct assessment for early childhood intervention:

1. To apply assessment practices that align with *evidence-based standards*
2. To apply assessment practices to fulfill specific early intervention *purposes*
3. To apply assessment practices to *reach data-driven decisions* about effective and high-quality services and supports for young children and families

Recommended standards for professional practice in assessment require that early interventionists make the following data-driven decisions for children: (1) determine which goals should be targeted through which interventions/services; (2) establish which children warrant different or more intensive interventions and when they should be implemented; and (3) determine in what ways programs and services at the local, state, and national levels should be improved (McLoughlin & Lewis, 1990; National Early Childhood Accountability Task Force, 2007).

We divide the chapter into two sections. Section one summarizes six general assessment practices that are required by national professional organizations and supported by emerging research. Section two describes recommended practices for three key decisions made by EI/ECSE professionals: *instructional planning, continuous performance monitoring*, and *accountability*. Several key terms are used throughout the chapter. Table 3.1 provides a summary of the key terms and associated definitions.

Table 3.1   Key Terms Used Throughout the Chapter

Key Term	Definition
Accountability	Accountability in public education refers to the "systematic collection, analysis, and use of information to hold schools, educators, and others responsible for the performance of students and the education system" (Education Commission of the States, 1998, p. 3).
Authentic assessment	Authentic assessment of young children refers to "the systematic recording of developmental observations over time about the naturally occurring behaviors and functional competencies of young children in daily routines by familiar and knowledgeable caregivers in the child's life" (Bagnato & Yeh Ho, 2006, p. 29).
Conventional testing	Conventional testing refers to "the administration of a highly structured array of testing tasks by an examiner in a contrived situation through the use of scripted examiner behaviors and scripted child behaviors in order to determine a normative score for purposes of diagnosis" (Bagnato, Neisworth, & Pretti-Frontczak, 2010).
Data-driven decision making	Data-driven decision making is a process by which teams design and revise instruction based upon authentic, comprehensive, valid, and reliable data.
Instructional planning	Instructional planning involves use of assessment information to identify children's strengths, emerging skills, and areas of need to then design appropriate instruction to enhance the child's learning experiences and developmental growth.
Performance monitoring	Performance monitoring is a recursive feedback process of adjusting and revising instruction in accordance with data that are systematically collected through ongoing observation and then documented, summarized, analyzed, and interpreted.

PROFESSIONAL PRACTICE STANDARDS FOR ASSESSMENT

Regardless of the assessment decision, there are recommended practices that must be understood and followed. In the United States, there are three sources for these recommended practices: professional organizations, various committee reports, and legislative policies, all of which influence how young children are assessed and families served.

Professional Organizations

The National Association for the Education of Young Children (NAEYC) and the Division for Early Childhood of the Council of Exceptional Children (DEC) are two major professional organizations in early childhood. Each of the professional organizations has produced specific, cross-referenced practice standards regarding assessment, curriculum, and program evaluation for all young children. These standards drive our daily work with children and families and must, similarly, drive state and national policies and practices to document the progress of children and the impact of programs. Specifically, NAEYC and DEC have produced, published, and updated collaborative documents on recommended assessment practice standards (DEC, 2007; NAEYC & National Association of Early Childhood Specialists in State Departments of Education [NAECS/SDE], 2003; Neisworth & Bagnato, 2005) that cover aspects of assessment relevant to infants, toddlers, and preschool children. These practice standards serve as the foundation for pre-service education of teachers and providers, for daily practice, and for certifying the quality of programs. Professional standards of practice in early childhood intervention distinguish the common and established values of our field, and they show an emerging applied evidence-base that validates adherence to their principles and practices.

Committee Reports

In recent years, summary reports have been published that have influenced the shape of assessment practices (National Academy of Sciences & National Research Council, 2008; National Early Childhood Accountability Task Force, 2007). The committees encompass researchers, policy makers, and practitioners. Their work, while at times controversial, provides input into how practices are identified and sometimes challenged.

Legislative Policies

Professional organizations and committee reports influence practices; however, it is legislation that most directly influences actual practice. The Individuals with Disabilities Education Act (IDEA) and No Child Left Behind (NCLB) are two pieces of federal legislation in the United States that help guide assessment practices. For example, NCLB, also called the Elementary Secondary Education Act, has as one of its goals to make every child "100% proficient" in state reading and math tests within 12 years. As a result, educators across states administer annual reading and math tests in grades three through eight.

A review of recommendations by professional organizations, committees, and legislation resulted in six common assessment themes. Recommendations include the use of assessment practices that are (1) authentic, (2) ongoing, (3) developmentally appropriate, (4) individualized, (5) natural, and (6) multi-factored. Table 3.2 illustrates how professional organizations, expert committees, and/or legislation promote each of the recommendations. Each recommended assessment practice is briefly described next.

#1: Authentic

The foundation for assessment should be to measure skills that demonstrate what the child is capable of doing in a real-world context (Bagnato, 2007). The word "authentic" refers to opportunities created for children that reflect typical experiences rather than discrete isolated tasks that are irrelevant to the child's daily life. For example,

Table 3.2 Policy Recommendations for Early Childhood Assessment Practices

Assessment Recommendations	DEC	NAE-YC	NECA-TF	NRC	IDEA	NCLB	Other
1. Authentic	X	X		X			
2. Ongoing	X	X	X	X	X	X	Head Start Bureau NASP
3. Developmentally Appropriate	X	X	X	X			Head Start Bureau NASDE NASP
4. Individualized	X	X	X	X	X	X	Head Start Bureau NASP
5. Natural	X	X	X	X	X		Head Start Bureau
6. Multi-factored	X	X	X	X	X	X	Head Start Bureau NASDE NASP

Key: DEC (Division for Early Childhood); IDEA (Individuals with Disabilities Education Act); NAEYC (National Association for the Education of Young Children); NASDE (National Association of State Directors of Special Education); NASP (National Association of School Psychologists); NCLB (No Child Left Behind); NECATF (National Early Childhood Accountability Task Force); NRC (National Research Council).

authentic assessment is creating opportunities for a child to demonstrate how they interact with a familiar caregiver, or how they act upon objects, versus asking a child to name pictures from a testing protocol or to tell a test administrator what can fly. Authentic assessment creates linkages between assessment and instructional/programmatic content and outcomes.

When we observe young children participating in authentic activities, we are observing the way they interact with people and their environment in ways that are useful and meaningful to them (Copple & Bredekamp, 2009; Neisworth & Bagnato, 2005). An authentic assessment process involves children performing activities that are functional in their everyday environments with familiar people.

#2: Ongoing

Assessment is an ongoing process, not a one-time observation. Assessment occurs across time and through multiple observations. Children are constantly changing and so is what they know, what they are learning, and what experiences they have had, all of which lead to new knowledge and skills. Therefore, it is necessary for the assessment of young children to be conducted over time to identify the latest thing that the child has learned, what is understood, and what is maintained (Copple & Bredekamp, 2009; DEC, 2007; Grisham-Brown, Hemmeter, & Pretti-Frontczak, 2005; NAEYC & NAECS/SDE, 2003).

Ongoing assessment occurs when a teacher constantly assesses the skills that a child has. In other words, a teacher continuously watches the children in his or her classroom to notice new abilities and to see where the child is in his or her development. According to the National Academy of Sciences (2008), there are ethical principles that educators must adhere to that underlie all assessment practices, making it necessary for teachers not to make decisions based solely on the basis of a single observation. In other words, so as to not deny a child services, educators must observe a child over and over in different settings to verify that they do or do not require special education services (NAEYC & NAECS/SDE, 2003).

#3: Developmentally Appropriate

Assessment practices should be developmentally appropriate for the child. Developmentally appropriate practice means that the assessment is suitable for the ages and dispositions of the children being assessed.

Considerations of culture, home language, poverty level, and ability level are important factors in the assessment of young children relative to developmental appropriateness (NAEYC & NAECS/SDE, 2003).

For example, an assessment is not appropriate for a child who speaks Spanish if the test was designed and field tested on all English-speaking children. DEC states that assessments should also be individually appropriate, which means that the suitability of the test for a student is determined by their personal characteristics, which *could* include factors like those specified by NAEYC—culture, home language, poverty level, and ability level (DEC, 2007).

#4: Individualized

The assessment should be individualized for all children. The assessment must be adaptable, especially for children who have functional limitations; moreover, assessments must be individualized for children who are developmentally delayed, at risk, and from culturally and/or linguistically diverse populations. Service providers should be able to assess the child on any level (e.g., a child with communication delay, a child with developmental delay). Adaptable, in terms of assessment, basically means that a service provider has the flexibility to make changes to the assessment to accommodate the needs of the child being assessed.

Individualization and adaptability of the assessment for children with special needs is a critical aspect of accommodating diverse learners which may include lengthening the amount of time for which a child has to answer, giving the assessors the flexibility to present the information verbally or show the child something, flexibility in how toys are used and demonstrated, and larger pictures and print sizes (DEC, 2007). Other modifications may include, but are not limited to, lessening the number of items, changing the criteria for how a task is to be performed, using a different tool to assess the child, or changing what the child has to do to demonstrate a skill. Providing individualized and specialized practices for children that need greater adaptations ensures that all children can participate and that none are held back from participating because they have a delay (DEC, 2007).

#5: Natural

Assessment must be a natural process in two ways—the use of structured observation as the preferred form of authentic assessment, and observation of each child doing typical things in their everyday settings and routines. Children are most comfortable in their typical setting and will typically perform to their highest capability in their comfort zone. Therefore, assessment should be done in a child's natural environment (Administration for Children, Youth and Families, 2000; Jackson, Pretti-Frontczak, Harjusola-Webb, Grisham-Brown, & Romani, 2009). Examples of familiar settings or natural situations include a child's classroom, at home, at the grocery store with a parent, on the playground, or at childcare (Neisworth & Bagnato, 2004). Assessment data must be gathered from a child's familiar setting to produce results that are reflective of a child's natural performance (NAEYC & NAECS/SDE, 2003). It makes no sense to test a child in a situation in which they are not perfectly familiar and comfortable (Bagnato, 2005).

Authentic assessment should also take place during a child's daily routines (DEC, 2007; NAEYC & NAECS/SDE, 2003; Pretti-Frontczak, Jackson, McKeen, & Bricker, 2008). According to Neisworth and Bagnato (2004), authentic assessment relies heavily on the observation of a child in his or her natural environment during routine happenings to yield results that show a child has had the opportunity to demonstrate his or her competencies in every way possible. For example, a child who goes to childcare each day may follow a strict schedule. This schedule of daily events may include being greeted by the teacher with a hug, playing in the block area with friends, having circle time, playing outside, using the restroom, going to lunch, and then having a nap. If the child does this routine daily, it becomes familiar, like clockwork, in the child's mind. The child begins to predict or understand what will happen next. It would be best for an assessor to collect data on this child in their typical routines to avoid disrupting their routines and learning environment.

#6: Multi-Factored

Assessment information is gathered from multiple sources and using multiple approaches. Early childhood professionals agree that data must be collected from multiple sources to be beneficial to the child, and to be considered a part of an authentic assessment. To gather information from multiple sources means to interview or collect information from people the child comes into contact with in the context of the child's routines. These people could include parents, grandparents, other relatives, foster parents, occupational therapists, speech pathologists, physical therapists, physicians, childcare workers, preschool teachers, Sunday school teachers, and others who are familiar with the child.

DEC (2007) encourages family-centered and team-based processes of assessment. Assessing a child in a team-based format creates opportunities for team members to collect data during a child's routine, across multiple settings, and using multiple measures. These team members may include a child's developmental interventionist, an early intervention consultant, a home visitor, or any type of therapist or physician. Examples of different ways of understanding child development and learning may include examining written artifacts such as pictures, art projects, writing samples, having conversations with individuals familiar with the child (e.g., family and caregivers), and assessing children in their daily classroom and school settings, which may include various activity centers, transitions between activities, free-choice play times, small group activities, meals, and outdoor play. A multi-modal approach leads to a better understanding of the child because of the richness of data that are gathered.

Recommended practices help create an infrastructure to reduce long-standing fragmentation of early childhood policies and practices in assessment. They are intended to aid in decision making. When effective assessment practices are used to assess a child, accurate information is used to make decisions about a child's early childhood program.

DATA-DRIVEN DECISION MAKING

Teachers make decisions on a regular basis. In fact, early research on teacher decision making and efficacy estimated that teachers made as many as 1,300 decisions daily (Jackson, 1968). At the heart of making data-driven decisions is the ability to gather and use information for an individual child and groups of young children. Three key decisions are reached by EI/ECSE professionals: (1) which child outcomes should be targeted through which interventions/services; (2) how children are responding to instructional efforts, and when children warrant different or more intensive intervention; and (3) how educational and developmental interventions at the program/state/federal level can be improved.

A five-step process is suggested to guide providers in making data-driven decisions, including gathering information, documenting, summarizing, analyzing, and interpreting data. The primary way information is *gathered* is through observation. Observation can be defined as a "rigorous act of examining a specific behavior of interest in the context of daily routines" (Johnson, LaMontagne, Elgas, & Bauer, 1998, p. 218). Observations allow early childhood educators to learn about children's interests, preferences, and styles of communication and interaction, as well as their strengths and emerging skills related to the general curriculum. Providers are then encouraged to *document* (i.e., record) children's performance using written narratives such as anecdotal notes, gathering permanent products such as writing samples or videos, and collecting counts and tallies (Grisham-Brown et al., 2005). It is not sufficient, however, to gather volumes of data if they are not used.

A necessary step to using data is *summarizing* using a mixture of narrative summaries, visual summaries, and numerical summaries. *Analyzing* data summaries is the fourth step, when one examines patterns and trends. Analysis can be done through visual inspection, comparison of standard scores to a normative group or criterion set forth in a measure, and/or through discussion with team members, where predictable actions by the children are recognized and their implications for development considered.

Lastly, providers need to *interpret* and make meaning out of the data. Interpretations should lead to decisions regarding who needs to learn what, whether certain outcomes are a higher priority than others, the type and level of instruction that is needed, and how and when to revise or change instructional efforts.

Instructional Planning

Planning instruction for young children has never been more challenging, particularly given the increased number of children with disabilities who are served in community settings and the overall diversity of the population of young children being served. Determining what to teach to whom and/or what level of instruction individuals and groups of children require can be a daunting task, particularly if providers rely on brief checklists that probe skill mastery or conventional tests.

Probes or checklists of mastery skills are problematic for a number of reasons. First, they tend to be dichotomous in nature—either the child demonstrates the skill, or they do not. Second, they are often organized into arbitrary developmental domains or content areas and by ages that, at best, have face validity—but rarely for children with disabilities. Third, they are often brief or may have only select items from a given area of development and may not fully assess a child's ability.

Conventional tests are equally problematic. First, most do not meet recommended practice standards and have no evidence base for use to accomplish specific early intervention purposes. Second, items and procedures are not matched to the objectives of most EI/ECSE programs and are often insensitive to gains made by children. Third, the reliance on standardized procedures results in biased, unfair, and inaccurate conclusions regarding a child's capabilities (i.e., a child's incapability to perform on scripted tasks is misrepresented as their inability). Fourth, test items lack functional content; items do not directly link to instructional efforts and may narrow curricular efforts.

Assessment practices that provide comprehensive information regarding a child's performance across interrelated areas of development and content, information regarding children's interests and preferences, and information regarding family priorities and concerns are needed. Table 3.3 summarizes the quality characteristics of a comprehensive approach to assessment and data-driven decision making for instructional planning

Table 3.3   Quality Characteristics of a Comprehensive Approach to Assessment

Assessment Component	Quality Characteristics
Comprehensive	• Assess all areas of development (e.g., motor, adaptive, cognitive, communication, social) • Assess all subject areas (e.g., language arts, science, social studies, math, technology, health) • Consider the interrelatedness of development • Gather information regarding strengths, emerging skills, and needs
Interests and Preferences	• Establish what motivates a child • Identify preferred activities, toys/materials, people, and actions • Establish what sustains a child's interest, participation, and engagement
Priorities and Concerns	• Obtain information from families and other familiar caregivers regarding a child's participation in daily routines and events • Discuss priorities for families and other familiar caregivers

Information from assessment for programming is systematically documented and summarized. Summaries should provide a complete picture of the child's current skills, abilities, knowledge, and preferences across daily activities and routines. From the summaries, teams can identify patterns or reoccurring trends that may require varying degrees and types of instruction. Specifically, from such assessment information, teams can interpret or make decisions regarding who needs to learn what and target meaningful outcomes that can be aligned to the appropriate instructional efforts. When serving groups of young children, teams will need to consider individual child patterns and trends as well as how groups of children are doing in terms of meeting common outcomes. Overall, quality instructional planning for individual and groups of children can be conceptualized as a tiered model allowing for differentiation and individualization.

Tiered models, which are not unique to EI/ECSE, often contain a bottom tier which includes common or universal outcomes and needs for all children, a second tier for targeted or temporary needs for some children, and a third tier for highly individualized needs. When planning instruction, providers will need to determine who needs to learn what, or rather identify needs for individuals and groups of children. The more experienced the provider, the more the process will become automatic; however, those who are new to the field may need to use a key part of their planning time (or secure planning time) to "sort" or identify children's needs.

Creating an image of a tiered model may help providers plan instruction and systematically identify children's needs. Thus, Figure 3.1 provides one example of a tiered model that can be used to plan and revise instruction based upon a child's needs. At the bottom tier, or Tier 1, are common or universal outcomes that all children need to learn. Tier 1 needs are derived from federal outcomes, state standards, and developmental milestones appropriate for a given age group. When a child's needs are identified as Tier 1, it means development and growth is considered on track. For example, all preschool-aged children should be learning how to participate in small group activities; use words, phrases, and sentences to inform, ask questions, and provide explanations; carry out all toileting needs; count objects; and engage in cooperative play with others. In Figure 3.1, counting is used and defined as a Tier 1 need to signify that all preschoolers are receiving instruction related to counting.

Depending upon the content/demands of the situation or where a child is in the learning cycle, they may experience difficulty with a

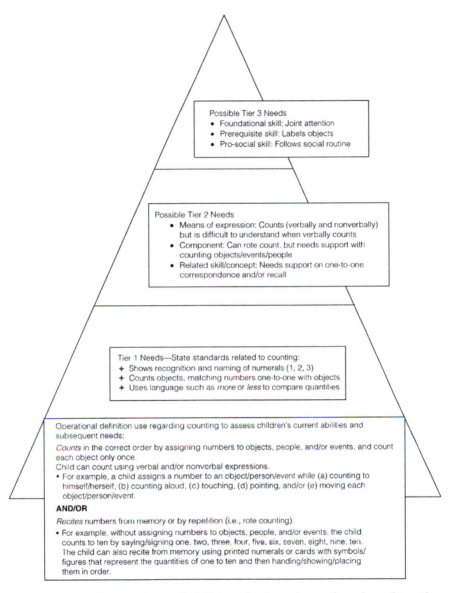

Figure 3.1 Illustration of children's tiered needs related to the common outcome of counting.

means of expression (e.g., saying, labeling, gesturing, manipulating, compiling), or with a component of a larger/more sophisticated concept or skill (e.g., has difficulty remaining with the group at story time, which is a component of participation). At other times, a child's progress may have stalled, or there is a related or concurrent skill that needs additional support for development and progress to continue. Whether a preschooler is struggling with a means of expression, missing a component of a larger skill/concept, or if their development has stalled, the child is demonstrating a Tier 2 need, meaning the child requires additional scaffolding/support for development and progress to continue. For example, a child may need additional support to remain in a group, to be understood by others, and/or to sequence while concurrently learning to count higher. Figure 3.1 again provides examples of Tier 2 needs related to the common outcome of counting, where a child counts repeatedly only to five and may need instruction on sequencing or recall to see further gains in counting higher or more. As teams determine whether a child has a true Tier 2 need, they should simultaneously consider whether quality Tier 1 instruction has been provided with fidelity, and whether the instruction was developmentally appropriate.

Tier 3 needs are where a child may be missing a foundational or prerequisite skill/concept that is keeping them from accessing, participating, and making progress toward common outcomes. For example, a child may tantrum every time they are asked to follow a social routine, lack joint attention or conversational turn-taking, or still may be working on reaching and grasping objects even though they are of preschool age. When a child is missing a foundational, prerequisite, or prosocial/age-appropriate skill, she is demonstrating a Tier 3 need. Figure 3.1 provides examples of possible Tier 3 needs that would increase a child's access, participation, and progress toward the common outcome of counting.

Once children's needs are identified, providers may find that several children, or even a single child, can have many Tier 2 and Tier 3 needs. Given the complexities of serving diverse children, it is impossible to provide the instruction required to address higher-tiered needs when numerous Tier 2 and 3 needs for multiple children have been selected. Thus, providers should prioritize in terms of where to begin instruction. When setting priorities for individual and groups of children, outcomes that are a priority for all team members and what the child needs to access, participate, and make progress in the classroom as well as outcomes that will benefit the child in the home and community should be discussed.

After deciding upon priorities for instruction, providers are ready to consider the type and frequency of instructional efforts to implement. The level of intensity and frequency of instruction should match the level of the child's need. For example, more individualized, intensive, and intentional instruction should be provided for a Tier 3 need. Providers should use a variety of evidenced-based instructional strategies (from nondirective to directive) again matching frequency and intensity with level of need. Revising initial instructional decisions in terms of their accuracy and efficacy (i.e., to determine if instructional efforts are promoting growth and development, leading to family satisfaction, and resulting in quality programming) is the next critical decision providers need to make.

Continuous Performance Monitoring

As stated in Table 3.1, performance monitoring is defined as a recursive feedback process of adjusting and revising instruction in accordance with data that are systematically collected through ongoing observation and then documented, summarized, analyzed, and interpreted. Once the needs of a child or a group of children have been identified and the appropriate instruction initiated, teams must engage in continuous performance monitoring to determine the impact and success of their instructional efforts and to revise or change as needed. The term "performance monitoring" over "progress monitoring" was chosen to impress upon teams the need to broadly describe and examine changes over time not only in terms of acquisition or mastery of skills, but also in more qualitative and holistic ways. For example, instead of relying on changes in test scores or a checklist that illustrates mastery of a skill to know whether a child is benefiting from instructional efforts, teams should also consider changes in levels of independence, consistency, frequency, and latency. Table 3.4 provides several examples of dimensions of behavior that should be considered when making decisions about a child's performance over time.

As with identifying children's needs and associated levels of instruction, performance-monitoring efforts should also be applied to a tiered approach. In other words, the frequency and intensity of data collection varies depending upon the child's needs and matched level of instruction. Figure 3.2 provides a depiction of performance monitoring within a tiered model. At Tier 1, teams are monitoring all children's performances toward common outcomes. As defined earlier, common outcomes are the standards and milestones expected for all children (regardless of ability) at a given age. Teams should monitor performance toward standards and developmentally appropriate milestones at least once a year, preferably (given the variability of young children's development) three or four

Table 3.4   Examples of Dimensions of Behavior

Dimension of Behavior	Examples of a Child's Performance
Frequency (number of times a Behavior occurs—how often)	• Number of times child initiates toileting each day • Number of times child manipulates objects with both hands during free play • Number of times child initiates greetings to peers during morning arrival • Number of successful transitions from one activity to another across the daily routine
Accuracy (how well a Behavior is demonstrated)	• Completes tasks without assistance • Talks without omitting or substituting particular sounds • Writes first name using upper- and lowercase letters that are recognizable • Correctly categorizes objects based upon their function
Latency (length of time to respond)	• Time between teacher verbal direction and child response • Time between when a visual cue is given a child makes a choice • Time between being asked a question and the child answering the question • Time between a high emotional response and child regaining composure to a more neutral response
Duration (how long a Behavior lasts or is demonstrated)	• How long a child participates in circle-time activity by remaining with the group, looking, and listening • How long a child cries after Mom leaves the classroom • How long a child works to complete puzzles • How long a child plays near peers
Endurance (how many times the behavior is repeated)	• Takes 10 steps • Communicates for two or more exchanges • Counts 10 objects • Remains seated for three minutes

times a year. Information regarding performance at Tier 1 can be obtained through the re-administration of a comprehensive and authentic assessment, often times through the re-administration of a curriculum-based assessment (CBA). Monitoring performance at Tier 1 is important to inform providers as to whether children's needs have changed since the beginning of the year, hence requiring a change in the frequency and intensity of instruction and/or what is being targeted. For example, when monitoring children's performance toward the common outcomes of counting, providers are encouraged to re-administer a CBA containing

Performance Monitoring

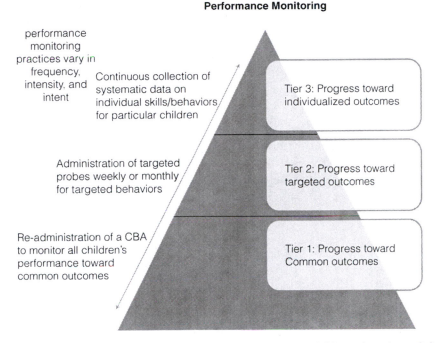

performance monitoring practices vary in frequency, intensity, and intent

Continuous collection of systematic data on individual skills/behaviors for particular children

Tier 3: Progress toward individualized outcomes

Administration of targeted probes weekly or monthly for targeted behaviors

Tier 2: Progress toward targeted outcomes

Re-administration of a CBA to monitor all children's performance toward common outcomes

Tier 1: Progress toward Common outcomes

Figure 3.2 Depiction of performance monitoring within a tiered model.

items related to counting near the beginning of the year, at a midpoint, and a few months before the end of the year. Re-administration of the CBA would be done with *all* children regardless of associated needs. In other words, the common outcome of counting would be monitored several times a year even for a child who initially had the Tier 3 need of joint attention as the foundational or perquisite skill needed to see progress toward the outcome of counting.

Within Tier 2, performance monitoring consists of more frequent and targeted efforts; however, not for all skills or for all children. In other words, at Tier 2, providers gather data on select groups of children who may have similar needs related to a component of a common outcome; a challenge with expressing themselves verbally or nonverbally as expected for their age, or even for a skill that has stalled and needs a boost of instruction to become more sophisticated and/or at a level expected. At Tier 2, data are collected perhaps as often as every week or a few times a month. Instructional efforts at Tier 2 should be considered temporary and in prevention of needing Tier 3 support; thus, sufficient and timely data are needed to quickly determine how the child is responding to more intense and more frequent instruction. Curriculum-based measures (i.e., standardized, short tests), re-administration of key parts of CBAs (at least CBAs with enough items to be sensitive to change), and/or the collection of anecdotal notes, written products, or rubrics can all be used at Tier 2; it is just a matter of being able to administer them more than a few times a year. For example, providers may track a group of children whose performance related to counting objects had stalled (i.e., they were able to count only five objects) on a related issue of sequencing. This means instruction was provided on a concurrent skill of sequencing and tracked weekly to see if progress with sequencing would have a positive impact on the children subsequently being able to count beyond five objects.

At Tier 3, data are collected under a rigorous schedule that would likely include daily and/or on given occurrences (e.g., following each conflict, during circle time). It is critical that data not only be collected more often at Tier 3, but with greater individualization and specificity, and that interpretations are made on a daily or weekly basis. Teams cannot wait until a parent-teacher conference or annual review of an individualized education plan to determine if their instructional efforts were aiding a child's increased access, participation, and progress. Closely monitoring performance allows providers to revise instruction routinely to assure the child is reaching their maximum potential. For example, providers may need to collect data during each transition for a child who was struggling with following a classroom routine, which was ultimately keeping the child from engaging in activities or completing tasks.

Accountability

Evaluating the overall impact and outcomes of early intervention programs using performance benchmarks is the third key data-driven decision. The accountability movement associated with NCLB has influenced EI/ECSE in the form of a downward extension of a "tests and testing" model employed by school-age programs. Advocates for young children, while proponents of accountability, are concerned that existing models are detrimental not only to children, but to their families and the programs and personnel who serve them. Much controversy surrounds the testing of infants, toddlers, and preschoolers, particularly those with disabilities and delays. While the early childhood intervention field supports, generally, the need to monitor the progress of young children in diverse programs, little agreement exists on how desired information should be obtained, who should collect the information, and perhaps most importantly, how the information should be summarized and interpreted. Moreover, there is a dearth of research on accountability assessment practices in early childhood intervention. Many of the current efforts are driven by K–12 models or, worse yet, appear to parallel earlier national accountability mandates under the National Reporting System (NRS) initiated by the Head Start Bureau (e.g., narrowing the scope of what is assessed and ultimately taught, distracting from other critical program needs, and linking test findings to funding allocations).

With increasing pressure, government agencies are requiring accountability data from programs serving young children (Harbin, Rous, & McLean, 2005). Many of the efforts, in the form of regulations, are being proposed and implemented without regard for professional "best practices," usefulness and benefits to children and families, and the glaring absence of research. In particular, state and federal outcome indicators are emerging to document accountability. Interdisciplinary professionals in the fields of early childhood intervention (i.e., public and private early care and education, Head Start, and early intervention) have an ethical and moral responsibility to advocate for assurances that sanctioned professional standards will be honored when measurement strategies for accountability are designed and mandated by state and federal entities.

While accountability methods and standards must meet professional standards, they must also be sensible and equitable. Policies must reflect the uniqueness and diversity of the EI/ECSE field (e.g., settings in which children spend time, education level of teachers) compared to school-aged children and the individual needs of its vulnerable young children and families. In the brief discussions below, we operationalize professional standards and relate them to what we believe should be "best practices" in accountability:

1. Young Children Are Individuals, so, Their Programs and Performance Data Must Be Individualized

The distinguishing characteristic of the field of early childhood intervention is that we focus on the strengths and needs of individual children rather than making broad group or age comparisons. At the base, intra-individual (occurring within a child; for example the same child over time) progress is the most important criteria for significant change, not inter-individual (occurring between children; for example, child to child) comparisons. Further, the more one aims to compare young children with differing abilities to a normative group, the less valid and trustworthy the conclusions; this fact makes accountability in early childhood, particularly for those children with disabilities, fundamentally different from school-age accountability standards. All young children should be entitled to individualized instruction that meets their unique learning needs. Even children who are at risk, English-language learners, or those with minor articulation concerns may require individualized programs, and their performance over time on family priorities must be the criteria for accountability. Thus, common outcomes should be universally acceptable for the diverse cultural, linguistic, and individual needs for all young children. Further, if individual performance is to be rated, documented, and then aggregated, the sum should be seen only as valid as its parts.

For children with disabilities, the goal of a programmatic intervention is not to ensure progress toward a typical level of functioning. Rather, parents and professionals seek to document performance toward individual goals and to alter pre-intervention developmental trajectories. For children with significant disabilities, maintenance of performance or prevention of regression, not progress, is the goal of the intervention. All young children deserve performance criteria and measurement methods that are sensible and equitable.

2. Accountability Data Cannot Be Interpreted in the Absence of Additional Information about the Child

A number of variables impact change in children's development and include prior exposure to intervention, regularity of participation and engagement in the program, and mediating factors (e.g., serious head injury between entry and exit data collection; uncontrolled seizure activity). As well, cultural expectations will impact behavioral changes in young children. Differing family ideas about when children should learn certain skills will likely impact how quickly children learn them. In addition, the age of the child must be considered. Younger children may show less apparent developmental delay than older children. Given the various ways in which change in child development can be affected, consideration should be given to defining progress for individual children. For some children with disabilities, developmental changes in some areas are realistic goals. For others, progress may be defined as not acquiring additional disabilities or not regressing in development.

3. Child Progress Data for Accountability Cannot Be Interpreted in the Absence of Data on the Program Itself

Aggregated data on changes in children's acquisition of developmental competencies or changes in trajectory are meaningless unless related to aggregated data about the programs and services in which children participate. There must be a functional interrelationship between each child's patterns of progress and the type, quality, length, and intensity of their programs and the type of teaching and care strategies used. As well, the role of program providers must be considered in the context of analyzing accountability data. The type and amount of educational background of program providers may impact their capacity to deliver high-quality interventions with fidelity sufficient to impact child change. Similarly, the consistency with which program providers collect data to measure child change must be considered (i.e., same provider collecting data; assessment fidelity). Larger program variables also have been found to affect change in children's development and should be considered when interpreting accountability data. These include the quality of the environment, the program's leadership, and family involvement in the program.

4. Developmentally Appropriate Accountability Data Must Be Used Only to Improve Program Quality and Practices, Not to Sanction Teachers or Their Programs

States are reforming their assessment and evaluation policies to meet the federal mandates for IDEA. Specifically, the child outcomes identified by the Office of Special Education Programs (OSEP) include (1) positive social emotional skills, including social relationships, (2) acquisition and use of knowledge and skills, and (3) use of appropriate behaviors to meet needs. For accountability purposes, program personnel are required to assess children's performance in these three areas near entry and again near exit (Hebbeler, Barton, & Mallik, 2008). Although state agencies have in place procedures for collecting accountability data following federal guidelines, the procedures are highly variable and generally unsubstantiated. For example, the legitimacy of interpreting children's performance with regards to the three OSEP child outcomes is open to question for at least two reasons.

First, each outcome is stated in broad language that makes valid and consistent measurement and comparison over time difficult if not impossible. That is, personnel, and the measures and procedures used, may define or conceptualize the three outcomes in very different ways. A cursory comparison of crosswalks that have been created between commonly used assessment instruments and OSEP outcomes indicates startling variability among the specific sets of assessment items that are aligned with each OSEP outcome. Second, measures or procedures for data collection have not been carefully delineated, nor have any measures or procedures been developed for said purpose or adequately tested. Using different measures and collecting information in different ways may lead to child change data that are simply not comparable either across children or for any given child over time.

The lack of empirical verification, in terms of both validity and reliability, for interpreting and operationalizing the outcomes and the categories is of extreme concern, because critical decisions may rest on accountability findings (i.e., future funding of Part C and 619 programs). Accountability data should represent *developmental performance*, not necessarily developmental progress. Thus, accountability data must not be used inappropriately as an excuse or punishment for professionals, their programs, agencies, or states supplying IDEA services to young children and their families. Safeguard procedures need to be implemented for states and programs that do not meet performance expectations. Individualized professional development and mentoring of teachers must be improved by making accountability data available to teachers and supervisors and by ensuring access to high-quality state technical assistance.

5. Metrics for Profiling Child Progress and Program Impact Must Be Sensitive to Small Increments of Individual Child Performances

Standard scores on conventional tests are not sensitive to individual patterns of progress in young children, especially those with disabilities and functional limitations. In contrast, metrics that compare each child's progress to his individual pre-intervention starting point are most sensitive to true progress (i.e., changes in performance over time). Such metrics include expected-actual developmental growth curves, goal-attainment scaling, number of curricular objectives achieved, increases or decreases in the frequency of particular behaviors, and number of skills displayed with and without prompts. Perhaps most important is the fact that progress metrics must focus upon tangible ultimate criterion standards such as the acquisition of functional competencies that improve independent life functioning, performance, and learning (e.g., walks independently), rather than dubious normative comparisons to nonrepresentative standardization samples (walks 15 steps across a balance beam going heel to toe).

CONCLUDING GUIDE-POINTS FOR DATA-DRIVEN DECISION MAKING "IN ACTION"

Early childhood interventionists balance many complementary and sometimes competing assessment responsibilities for young children with developmental disabilities. Assessment in everyday environments is the "key" component for executing these responsibilities and making a series of critical decisions underlying actions for the benefit of vulnerable children and families. In this chapter, we described six general assessment practices required by national professional organizations and supported by emerging research. We then detailed three "linked" assessment activities that are critical "keys" to effective and high-quality early intervention for our most vulnerable young children; that is, the application of assessment practices for (1) instructional planning, (2) performance monitoring, and (3) accountability. We conclude with several summative guide-points for applying data-driven decision making "in action" to link these three assessment activities so that they operate as a seamless and circular process of checks and balances.

- *Rely upon authentic assessment measures and observational processes.* By using authentic assessments, EI/ECSE professionals will both comply with best practices in the field and apply methods that ensure compatible functional content for assessment and instruction. Authentic assessments enable professionals to observe and prompt children's typical capabilities in everyday settings and routines in a natural rather than contrived process.
- *Select a uniform and dense curriculum of functional skills for children in your program.* Best practice presumes that administrators and early childhood intervention professionals will collaborate to choose a functional curriculum that matches the program's philosophy and the capabilities and needs of children in the program. Comprehensive and sequential curricula ensure continuity from birth to the transition at kindergarten. Sequential developmental and

functional content allows professionals and parents to align their authentic observational assessments with the appropriate content within the curricula to create individualized instructional objectives, intervention strategies, and plans that promote child progress. The alignment of assessment and instruction through the curriculum forms the basis for monitoring performance and modifying instruction so that efficacious programs are produced and continuous quality improvement is assured.

• *Align the content of the assessment, the curriculum, and the state and federal benchmarks for program success as the foundation for sensible accountability.* Too often, state and federal benchmarks and indicators used to evaluate child progress are divorced from programmatic content and common sense. Early childhood interventionists and administrators can advocate best for their children and the sustainability of their programs by promoting curriculum-referenced forms of authentic measurement. The developmental and functional content of curricula can be cross-walked with the indicators of success for children contained in state and federal performance standards. These linkages between curriculum content and standards can ensure sensible, sensitive, and synchronized targets for both children and programs.

References

Bagnato, S. J. (2005). The authentic alternative for assessment in early intervention: An emerging evidence-based practice. *Journal of Early Intervention, 28*(1), 17–22. doi:10.1177/105381510502800102

Bagnato, S. J. (2007). *Authentic assessment for early childhood intervention: Best practices.* New York: Guilford Press.

Bagnato, S. J., Neisworth, J., & Pretti-Frontczak, K. (2010). *LINKing authentic assessment and early childhood intervention: Best measures for best practices* (2nd ed.). Baltimore: Paul H. Brookes.

Bagnato, S. J., & Yeh-Ho, H. (2006). High-stakes testing with preschool children: Violation of professional standards for evidence-based practice in early childhood intervention. *KEDI Journal of Educational Policy, 3*(1), 23–43.

Copple, C., & Bredekamp, S. (Eds.) (2009). *Developmentally appropriate practice in early childhood programs* (3rd ed.). Washington, DC: National Association for the Education of Young Children.

Division for Early Childhood. (2007). *Promoting positive progress outcomes for children with disabilities: Recommendations for curriculum, assessment, and program evaluation.* Missoula, MT: Author.

Education Commission of the States. (1998). *Designing and implementing standards-based accountability systems.* Denver, CO: Author.

Grisham-Brown, J. L., Hemmeter, M. L., & Pretti-Frontczak, K. (2005). *Blended practices for teaching young children in inclusive settings*. Baltimore: Paul H. Brookes.

Harbin, G., Rous, B., & McLean, M. (2005). Issues in designing state accountability systems. *Journal of Early Intervention, 27*(3), 137–164. doi:10.1177/105381510502700301

Head Start Bureau. (1992). *Head Start program performance standards*. DHHS Publication No. ACF92-31131. Washington, DC: Department of Health and Human Services.

Hebbeler, K., Barton, L. R., & Mallik, S. (2008). Assessment and accountability for programs serving young children with disabilities. *Exceptionality, 16*(1), 48–63. doi:10.1080/09362830701796792

Jackson, P. W. (1968). Life in classrooms. New York: Holt, Rinehart, & Winston.

Jackson, S., Pretti-Frontczak, K., Harjusola-Webb, S., Grisham-Brown, J., & Romani, J. M. (2009). Response to intervention: Implications for early childhood professionals. *Language, Speech, and Hearing Services in Schools, 40*(4), 424–434. doi:10.1044/0161-1461 (2009/08-0027)

Johnson, L., LaMontagne, M., Elgas, P., & Bauer, A. (1998). *Blending early childhood and early childhood special education practices: Collaboration to meet the needs of children and their families*. Baltimore: Paul H. Brookes.

McLean, M., Wolery, M., & Bailey, D. B. (2004). *Assessing infants and preschoolers with special needs* (3rd ed). Columbus, OH: Pearson.

McLoughlin, J. A., & Lewis, R. B. (1990). *Assessing students with special needs* (4th ed). Columbus, OH: Merrill.

Meisels, S. J. (2000). Readiness and relationships: Issues in assessing young children, families, and caregivers. *Head Start Bulletin, 69*, 5–6. Retrieved from http://eclkc.ohs.acf.hhs.gov/hslc/Professional%20Development/Organizational%20Development/Cultivating%20a%20Learning%20Organization/FINAL-EHS.pdf

National Academy of Sciences & National Research Council. (2008). *Early childhood assessment: Why, what, and how?* Committee on Developmental Outcomes and Assessments for Young Children (C. E. Snow & S. B. Van Hemel, Eds.). Board on Children, Youth and Families, Board on Testing and Assessment, Division of Behavioral and Social Sciences and Education. Washington, DC: National Academies Press.

National Association for the Education of Young Children & National Association of Early Childhood Specialists in State Departments of Education (NAEYC & NAECS/SDE). (2003). *Early childhood curriculum, assessment and program evaluation: Building an effective and accountable system in programs for children birth to 8 years of age*. Washington, DC: NAEYC.

National Early Childhood Accountability Task Force. (2007). *Taking stock: Assessing and improving early childhood learning and program quality*. Pew Charitable Trusts. Retrieved from http://www.pewtrusts.org/uploadedFiles/wwwpewtrustsorg/Reports/Pre-k_education/task_force_report1.pdf

Neisworth, J. T., & Bagnato, S. J. (2004). The mismeasure of young children: The authentic assessment alternative. *Infants and Young Children, 17*(3), 198–212.

Neisworth, J. T., & Bagnato, S. J. (2005). DEC recommended practices: Assessment. In S. Sandall, M. L. Hemmeter, B. F. Smith, and M. McClean (Eds.), *DEC recommended practice: A comprehensive guide for practical application in early intervention/early childhood special education* (pp. 45–70). Longmont, CO: Sopris West.

Pretti-Frontczak, K., Jackson, S., McKeen, L., & Bricker, D. (2008). Supporting quality curriculum frameworks in early childhood programs. In A. Thomas & J. Grimes (Eds.), *Best practices in school psychology V* (pp. 1249–1259). Washington, DC: National Association of School Psychologists; Texas: Psychological Corporation.

Chapter 4

Children with Disabilities, School Readiness, and Transition to Kindergarten

Sharon E. Rosenkoetter, Cristian M. Dogaru,
Beth Rous, and Carol Schroeder

Starting kindergarten is a major life experience for most children in developed countries around the world. In the United States, not all states require kindergarten enrollment; nevertheless, about 98 percent of children attend kindergarten in public or private schools, full day or half day, prior to their first-grade year (Zill, 1999). Kindergarten is popularly viewed as the beginning of the school experience in communities across the United States. Kindergarten is the time and place where all children are first asked to demonstrate for the record the competencies that will support their formative educational years and the course of their future lives (Mangione & Speth, 1998; Pianta & Cox, 1999; Pianta & Kraft-Sayre, 2003).

While transition to kindergarten may be anticipated with anxiety, excitement, and stress by children and their families, for the great majority, the emotions of this time have little noted impact on later development (Fowler, Schwartz, & Atwater, 1991; Wolery, 1999). Most children with and without disabilities adjust over time to changes in their environments from what they experienced during the prekindergarten years: the larger class size, the unfamiliar school building, different people, a more demanding curriculum, altered expectations, and new interactions and relationships (Carta & Atwater, 1990; Fowler et al., 1991; Vail & Scott, 1994).

For some children, however, especially those with special needs, the transition to kindergarten presents challenges in adjustment to school and, too often, limited success at mastering the school's demands (O'Brien, 1991). Such negative outcomes are ones that families, service providers, and community planners strive to avoid (Pianta & Walsh, 1996; Rous & Hallam, 2006). Even though many children with identified disabilities have already participated in early intervention and/or early childhood special education through the public school system, and even though most of the families of these children have previously interacted with personnel employed by school districts, research shows that families of young children with disabilities still view transition to kindergarten as a monumental event (Rosenkoetter & Rosenkoetter, 2001). The same is true for children and families at risk for school difficulties due to poverty (SERVE, 1998). Patterns of friendship and mentorship, attendance, class groupings, and teacher-child interaction during the early months of kindergarten affect achievement (Ladd, 2006; O'Connor & McCartney, 2007; Rist, 1970) and are likely to continue on into the elementary school years. Of course, these can be modified by future events including decisions by parents and teams that guide children's school programs.

This chapter will define transition and school readiness and offer two conceptual models for understanding them. The chapter will summarize transition research findings and describe current research. Finally, it will suggest key principles for families and practitioners and describe emerging trends and future directions. We hope that the work described here will aid services to children with disabilities and their families and prompt new research to support them at the pivotal point of kindergarten entry.

WHAT IS TRANSITION?

Transition to kindergarten may be defined as the process of moving children and their families from the prekindergarten environment of home, preschool, child care, or Head Start into a kindergarten setting (Bruder & Chandler, 1996; Head Start, 1989). This change process is multi-faceted, involving new roles for children, families, and service providers as well as altered expectations for their daily interactions and long term planning (Bruder & Chandler, 1996; Ramey & Ramey, 1994, 1998; Rosenkoetter, Hains, & Fowler, 1994; Rous & Hallam, 2006).

For children with disabilities and their families, transition to kindergarten is likely to be more complex than for typically developing children. Due to their disabilities, children with special needs may experience the new environment differently from their typically developing peers (Carta & Atwater, 1990; Katims & Pierce, 1995), and their parents are more likely to worry about both the details of each day and the long-term outcomes of the process (Rosenkoetter & Rosenkoetter, 2001). In addition to a classroom teacher and perhaps an educational assistant, children with disabilities may have a number of therapists, other service providers, and administrators. Transition to kindergarten thus may mean leaving the prekindergarten set of familiar service providers and coming to understand and trust another group of professionals whose policies and practices are likely to differ (Wolery, 1999). Transition requires considerable new learning on the part of both children with disabilities and their parents.

WHAT IS SCHOOL READINESS?

The concept of readiness for kindergarten has received growing attention from policy makers, educators, parents, and researchers as it has become clear that children who struggle initially in kindergarten often continue to be challenged during their later school years (Task Force on School Readiness, 2005). As a result of difficulties in school, many youth drop out of high school and are unable to compete in a society that demands increasing literacy, numeracy, and social skills. Further, the rate of failure to complete secondary school is much higher among students from certain racial, ethnic, and geographic populations, including students with disabilities (U.S. Department of Education [USDOE], 2009; USDOE, OSERS, 2006).

Various professionals disagree on a definition of school readiness, stressing different elements and emphasizing different academic and social skills. The definition that one adopts leads to varying approaches to assessment and intervention with children at risk and guides program standards. Curricula in preschool and kindergarten are also developed based on the adopted definition of readiness. There are three primary approaches to the concept of school readiness.

First Approach: Focus on the Child as Ready or Not Ready

Many elements of the discourse about readiness have focused on the young child's developmental maturity (Ilg, Ames, Haines, & Gillespie, 1978) or skill preparation (Head Start, n.d.) for the tasks that kindergarten will present. For example, Kagan, Moore, and Bredekamp (1995), writing on behalf of the National Education Goals Panel, defined the five dimensions for children's early development and learning that the Panel viewed as the foundations for school readiness: (1) physical well-being and motor development, (2) social and emotional development, (3) approaches toward learning, (4) language development, and (5) cognition and general development. Many approaches to fostering child development, such as that espoused by the Goals Panel itself, have also stressed the importance of children's access to high-quality preschool education, supportive parenting, and essential nutrition and health care to facilitate school readiness and later academic success (USDOE, 1991).

During recent years, movements to increase accountability for performance outcomes swept through the business sector, state and federal government, and K–12 education. States and programs then began to shift this emphasis to early care and education (Hebbeler & Barton, 2007). Head Start identified a set of learning outcomes expected for children who completed its programs (Head Start, n.d.). Individual states developed or adopted early learning standards, guidelines, or benchmarks to define clearly what young children should know and do at specific ages or upon entry to kindergarten (Scott-Little, Kagan, & Frelow, 2005; Scott-Little, Kagan, Frelow, & Reid, 2008).

The downward extension of curriculum and academic expectations from elementary school to kindergarten has exacerbated the child-focused understanding of school readiness (Kemp & Carter, 2000). Growing numbers of parents are waiting a year to send their 5-year-old children to kindergarten (Deming & Dynarski, 2008); now one in six children enters kindergarten at age 6, not 5, a practice known as *academic redshirting*. Increasing numbers of school districts have experimented with various types of transition classes for children who were judged to be not ready for either kindergarten or first grade (Gredler, 2006; Mantzicopoulos, 2003). Local policies on retention in kindergarten for children considered unready for first grade continue to vary from place to place and from year to year (Frey, 2005). States have tinkered with their legal age for school entry in efforts to make all children "ready" for kindergarten (Stipek, 2002). In response to all these efforts, the National Association for the Education of Young Children, the nation's largest professional organization for early childhood personnel, adopted and continues to uphold a position statement on school readiness that opposes redshirting, transition classes, and retention and advocates a broader view of school readiness that is more in line with the definitions to be discussed below (1990; revised 1995).

Second Approach: Focus on the Setting and Social Construction of Readiness

Graue (1993), a former kindergarten teacher, observed that the same child could be ready, very ready, or not at all ready for kindergarten, depending upon the specific kindergarten in which the child enrolled. Her research findings challenged the within-the-child, ready/not ready conception of school readiness. Data from the National Center for Education Statistics (2009) supported an obvious conclusion: Not all children have the same opportunities to develop foundational learning skills prior to school entry, and accordingly, they arrive at kindergarten with different levels of competencies that facilitate school learning. According to Graue's pioneering research, readiness is an idea that is socially constructed by parents, teachers, and children as they interact and compare children's skill level in their schools, neighborhoods, and communities.

Subsequent discussions led to the notion of *Ready Schools* (National Education Goals Panel, 1998), which posited that the school (i.e., the kindergarten setting) must make itself ready to address the skill levels of any children who enroll. The document outlined 10 "keys to ready schools" that resulted in numerous educational change initiatives:

1. Smooth the transition between home and school
2. Strive for continuity between early care and education programs and elementary schools
3. Help children learn and make sense of their complex and exciting world
4. Be committed to the success of every child
5. Be committed to the success of every teacher and every adult who interacts with children during the school day
6. Introduce or expand approaches that have been shown to raise achievement
7. Exist as learning organizations that alter practices and programs if they do not benefit children
8. Serve children in communities
9. Take responsibility for results
10. Have strong leadership (p. 5)

This philosophy of readiness fits well with the growing diversity of American schools, in that a rapidly increasing percentage of young children speak a language other than standard English at home

(*Education Week*, 2004, citing the U.S. Bureau of Citizenship and Immigration Services, 2001). The Ready Schools philosophy is also congruent with inclusion in the least restrictive environment for children with disabilities, even if a child lacks certain normative achievements (Turnbull, Turnbull, & Wehmeyer, 2007).

Third Approach: Combination of Approaches One and Two

In its purpose statement, the No Child Left Behind Act of 2001 blended the two previous understandings of school readiness: First, the law required a series of actions, including "challenging State academic standards so that students, teachers, parents, and administrators can measure progress against common expectations for student academic achievement" (Sec. 1001[1]). Second, it required schools to meet

> the educational needs of low achieving children in our Nation's highest-poverty schools, limited English proficient children, migratory children, children with disabilities, Indian children, neglected or delinquent children, and young children in need of reading assistance. (Sec. 1002 [2])

The stated intent of this complex, demanding, and controversial law is that "all children have a fair, equal, and significant opportunity to obtain a high-quality education" (Sec. 1001 Introduction). Stated otherwise, the aim is that all children become ready to profit from the instruction offered in elementary school and to build a foundation for later school success. A smooth transition for young children from home and prekindergarten programs into kindergarten is a part of developing that readiness.

Results-based accountability has led to a greater emphasis on assessing individual young children to identify their school readiness, age-expected functioning, or achievement of early learning guidelines or standards. Program evaluations and ongoing systems for assessment of children's functioning and school readiness are being implemented to determine the need for changes in specific programs and funded activities to promote successful outcomes (Hebbeler, Barton, & Mallik, 2008). Although there is widespread agreement about the benefits of a well-coordinated system (Rous, LoBianco, Moffett, & Lund, 2005), states vary considerably in the extent to which early learning standards, assessments, and program evaluations are compatible, coordinated, or operative in the daily work of teachers and administrators (National

Early Childhood Accountability Task Force, 2007). How states coordinate the readiness monitoring of children with disabilities with other early childhood accountability efforts varies considerably (Harbin, Rous, & McLean, 2004). This process is highly uneven, as states continue to progress in their approaches to school readiness.

The National Governor's Association (NGA) has provided guidance for the states through its Task Force on School Readiness (2005). While it emphasized the importance of state, community, and family actions, the NGA report also stressed the goal of giving individual children the foundations that they need to be ready for school. Among its other recommendations to promote readiness, the Task Force charged states to "support schools, families, and communities in facilitating the transition of young children into the kindergarten environment" (p. 6). The highest levels of the educational community have linked the importance of transition planning and practices to supporting school readiness.

CONCEPTUAL MODELS OF TRANSITION

Two conceptual frameworks may help readers understand the relationships among the complex elements of transition that reflect its ecology, influence individual children's readiness and adjustment, and promote ongoing family involvement in their children's learning.

The Ecological and Dynamic Model of Transition

Pianta and Walsh (1996) proposed the Contextual Systems Model (CSM), which built on the Developmental Systems Theory as elucidated by Ford and Lerner (1992). CSM emphasizes the frames of culture and history for child development and views transition to kindergarten as a complex system of systems that develops and changes continuously across time. CSM evolved into the Ecological and Dynamic Model of Transition (EDMT; Rimm-Kaufman & Pianta, 2000). Among its systems are the transactive family/child system, peer/child system, teacher/child system, and neighborhood/child system. Each of these systems is embedded within the larger system of the preschool and the larger system of the kindergarten. Figure 4.1 illustrates the EDMT.

EDMT views transition as synergistic in that it is more than the sum of the interactions between subordinate systems. Over time, the

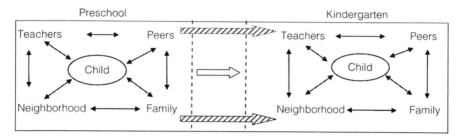

Figure 4.1   The ecological and dynamic model of transition (Rimm-Kaufman & Pianta, 2000).

interactions among transition system components form patterns, create expectations, and ideally grow in quality from their initial encounters. For example, prior to specific planning for the child's kindergarten entry, an important relationship has already developed between the prekindergarten system and the family/child system, and this relationship typically influences transition planning. When parents of young children with disabilities become involved with prekindergarten and kindergarten personnel in planning their child's transition to kindergarten, this new trilateral relationship comes to influence other systems, such as kindergarten teacher/child, kindergarten teacher/parent, kindergarten parent/other kindergarten parent, and kindergarten child/kindergarten child (Eccles & Harold, 1996; Hoover-Dempsey & Sandler, 1997; Smith, Connel, Wright, Sizer, & Norman, 1997). What is important is not only the development of these relationships, but also their characteristics, quality, and quantity. Various factors influence the strength of the developing relationships: for example, the parents' socioeconomic status, their educational and personal resources, the school's collaboration and communication with the family and other service providers, and community and cultural norms (Dogaru, 2008; Pianta & Walsh, 1996).

Thus, the transition to kindergarten is not a single event on a particular day, but rather, it is a process negotiated among the child, the family, the school system, the prekindergarten program(s), the community, and various individuals associated with each of these (Pianta & Cox, 1999; Rosenkoetter, Hains, & Fowler, 1994; Rous & Hallam, 2006). This negotiation is a process that requires time for planning and monitoring, the presence of communication structures to inform participants and promote relationships, preparation rituals to ready the child and family for kindergarten, and shared commitment to nurture the individual child and family. In the EDMT model, the family-child system is the constant. It moves from active participation with the prekindergarten teachers' and therapists' system to relationship building with the kindergarten personnel system. Importantly, the model emphasizes that all participants play significant roles in the nature and outcomes of the child's transition to kindergarten.

The National Early Childhood Transition Center Model

The following conceptual approach was developed by the National Early Childhood Transition Center (NECTC), which is the source of recent transition research related to young children with disabilities. By emphasizing both between-system and within-system dynamics, the NECTC model was proposed to demonstrate specific elements of effective transition and to define the outcomes that should be anticipated from successful transition (Harbin, Rous, Peeler, Schuster, & McCormick, 2007; Rous, Hallam, Harbin, McCormick, & Jung, 2007). Figure 4.2 demonstrates the dynamic context within which early childhood transition occurs, specifying its interactive elements but giving special attention to defining the state and community policies and relationships that are critical to the transition experiences of individual children with disabilities and their families.

Figure 4.3 illustrates the three critical characteristics in an interagency service system that effectively facilitates transition: (1) alignment and continuity, (2) supportive infrastructure, and (3) communication and relationships. This interagency system for transition influences and is influenced by the service policies and practices of local sending (prekindergarten) and receiving (kindergarten) programs, as together they shape the transition's outcomes over time: child preparation for kindergarten and child adjustment to kindergarten as well as family preparation for the transition to kindergarten and family adjustment to the new school. Each of these four areas of activity includes specific desired outcomes that can serve to guide the planning of supports that are provided during the transition process and that lead to the desired long-term outcomes: child success in school, and family engagement and involvement. Each element is affected by and must be responsive to other elements, but child and family remain the focus of the complex system (see Research Brief at http://www.hdi.uky.edu/SF/NECTC/Publications/resbriefs.aspx for additional explanation).

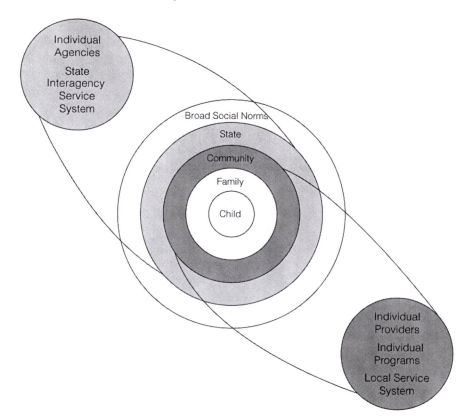

Figure 4.2   Context for transition to kindergarten (Rous, Hallam, Harbin, McCormick, & Jung, 2007).

Similarities across the Two Models

The same supersystems involved in transition to kindergarten are noted in both the EDMT Model and the NECTC Model: the prekindergarten and the kindergarten, with subsystems of family, peers, teacher (s), and the community, all focusing on the child. Both models emphasize the interactions between the supersystems and among the subsystems. Recommended practices for facilitating the transition to kindergarten of children with disabilities address all these factors as well (see Rous, 2008). Research has shown that the desired long-term results of effective transition as noted by the NECTC Model, namely child learning and parent involvement, are both predictors and outcomes for successful education (Love, Logue, Trudeau, & Thayer, 1992; O'Connor & McCartney, 2007; Pianta & Cox, 1999; Pianta &

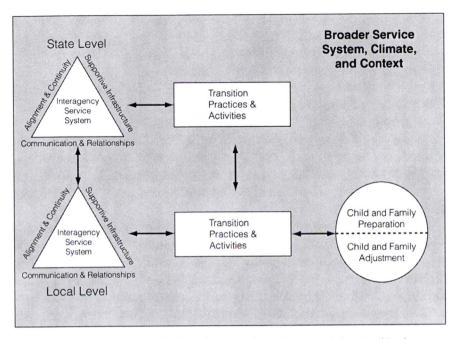

Figure 4.3   NECTC model for interactions in transition to kindergarten (Rous, Hallam, Harbin, McCormick, & Jung, 2007; Harbin, Rous, Peeler, Schuster, & McCormick, 2007).

Kraft-Sayre, 2003; Ramey & Ramey, 1994). The two models can help practitioners and researchers to organize existing research findings, identify gaps in knowledge, and foster coherent thinking about next steps in research and practice.

THE KNOWLEDGE BASE ABOUT SUCCESSFUL TRANSITION TO KINDERGARTEN

A great deal more is known today than 20 years ago about effective transitions for young children with disabilities and their families. Policy, research, and practice related to this issue have advanced in recent years. Most research and recommendations related to the transition of young children with disabilities to kindergarten evolved from numerous and widespread federal and state demonstration projects, technical assistance, and program evaluations in the 1980s and 1990s as well as from the reflections of parents, practitioners, and administrators about contemporary policies (Rosenkoetter, Whaley, Hains, & Pierce, 2001).

Since 1991, specific federal policies have guided the transition of toddlers from early intervention to preschool (Individuals with Disabilities Education Improvement Act of 2004 [IDEA, 2004]). The U.S. Department of Education (USDOE) continues to require policies related to transition at age 3 in each State Performance Plan (SPP). There is no federal legislation prescribing specific practices for the kindergarten transition for young children with disabilities except in Head Start (2003), which does serve more than 100,000 children with disabilities every year. Nevertheless, the federal provisions for children with disabilities leaving early intervention at age 3 have offered a prototype of effective practices for other ages as well, notably for the transition to kindergarten.

There has long been agreement that transition to kindergarten is a process that requires time, planning, written agreements, and commitment from relevant partners (Fowler, 1982; Head Start, 1989; Lazzari, 1991; Pianta & Cox, 1999; Rosenkoetter, Hains, & Fowler, 1994; Rous & Hallam, 2006). Hundreds, perhaps thousands, of advisory articles and state and local guidebooks have been circulated to support and operationalize these concepts (Rosenkoetter et al., 2001). Thousands of communities have grappled with the intent of federal and state policies and have developed local approaches to scaffold their transition efforts with families, yet transition dilemmas raised by the situations of individual children, families, and communities continue to reveal policy and implementation gaps (Harbin, Rous, Gooden, & Shaw, 2008). The continuing challenges appear to reflect the multi-agency, multilevel nature of transition as reflected in the complexity portrayed in the two models presented above.

Further, IDEA (2004) requires the use of a research base to guide all actions intended to support children and youth with disabilities. Section 635(a)(2) of IDEA underscores the need for services (by implication, including transition planning) to be grounded in scientifically based research "to the extent practicable." What, then, does research support regarding transition practices for young children with disabilities and their families?

NECTC Literature Review

A growing body of evidence defines and supports recommended practices. Although reviews of the early childhood transition literature have been included in advisory guides, no comprehensive review of the empirical research across early childhood transition points and populations has appeared in print. Thus, one of the major goals of the National Early Childhood Transition Center (NECTC) was to examine and synthesize existing research related to early childhood transition. NECTC staff searched for transition literature regarding children, both with and without disabilities, or their families. Articles reviewed were published from January 1990 to March 2006 and (1) were research based, (2) had appeared in major refereed journals, and (3) related to the early childhood years, birth to age 8. Since transition strategies for one group might help to inform practice for other groups, the articles concerned typically developing children, those at risk for developmental challenges, and those focusing on children with disabilities and their families. For the methodology, detailed findings, and resulting recommendations from this comprehensive literature search, see Rosenkoetter et al. (2008), which is available on the Internet.

As a result of this process, 50 articles from 29 different journals that met the criteria for inclusion in the review were drawn from 786 nominations. Of these 50 articles, 30 reported findings on the transition to kindergarten, with 19 studying children and 11 focusing on families. Eight of the child-focused studies related to children with disabilities, and four of the family-focused articles reported on families of children with disabilities.

Authors of this literature review noted their surprise at the paucity of empirical research on transition and the very limited number of studies that included more than 50 percent persons of color or second language learners. Two studies specifically addressed issues of children with significant disabilities and/or their families in transition, even though children with significant impairments elicit more concern related to the complexities of transition than do either typically developing children or those with mild impairments (Rosenkoetter & Rosenkoetter, 2001). It was noteworthy that the majority of studies on children with disabilities or their families had been published before 2002.

The authors of the NECTC review had planned to synthesize validated practices related to young children with disabilities in transition and to produce from this review a comprehensive list of validated recommendations for the field. These aims became impossible to achieve based on these past articles alone, because, as the authors noted, the majority of studies were correlational or descriptive rather than experimental in design. Nevertheless, some transition practices had sufficient support across the early childhood years, birth to age 8, to be recommended.

Conclusions from Child-Focused Studies

Based on the transition literature review and using the *Extent of Evidence Categorization Scheme* (What Works Clearinghouse, 2008), several findings were supported by sufficient investigation to receive a rating of moderate/large evidence. Such a rating requires more than one study on the topic, the participation of more than one program or school in the study, and a total sample size of at least 350 children across the studies. Following are findings supported by a moderate/large extent of evidence:

1. High-quality child care and developmentally appropriate preschool and kindergarten classrooms are associated with better academic outcomes, work habits, and social adjustment for children in their next school environments. This was true for children who were developing typically and for low-income, minority, urban children (five studies). Some participants in these studies were enrolled in Head Start, which includes children with disabilities and requires transition preparation activities.
2. Certain ecological factors, including higher socioeconomic status and income level, fewer family risk factors, better quality of neighborhood, and greater parent/school involvement and satisfaction, are associated with children's higher academic achievement and more positive social outcomes through the early elementary grades (three studies, none focused on disability).
3. A positive teacher-child relationship during transition to and in the next environment is associated with better cognitive outcomes for children who are developing typically as well as for those at risk. Such a positive teacher-child relationship also correlated with decreased externalizing behavior and positive social relationships for typically developing children (two studies, neither focused on disability).
4. Preschool and kindergarten teachers and their administrators said that they view social development and social communication skills (for example, expresses wants, takes turns, follows directions) as being more important for school readiness than academic skills (two studies, neither focused on disability).
5. Dissonance between the sending and receiving environments correlates with less successful transitions both for children who are developing typically and for those with developmental delays (two studies, one including children with disabilities).

Teaching children the skills to meet requirements in the next environment (sometimes referred to as "survival skills"; Rule, Feichtl, & Innocenti, 1990) is associated with more successful adjustment and positive outcomes after transition for young children with disabilities, developmental delays, or who are at risk for school failure (six studies, most focused on disabilities).

The NECTC reviewers also noted studies with promising practices related to children in transition. These four findings are strongly suggestive, though they do not meet the moderate/large evidence criteria listed above:

1. Demographic factors may hinder the child's initial adjustment in the next environment; e.g., rural setting, discrepancy between non-minority teachers and minority populations, or the child's initial lack of friends after transition (two studies, neither focused on disability).
2. Use of more transition practices at the beginning of the child's transition year may promote increased parent-initiated school involvement as well as higher academic achievement later in the year, especially for children in low and middle socioeconomic groups (one study, not focused on disability).
3. Providing transition assistance (health and family support services, parent involvement, curricular modifications) for an extended period of time upon entering a school system may prevent children at risk from being diagnosed with a developmental disability in the elementary grades (one study, participants did not have identified disabilities initially).
4. Although adequate preparation for skills needed in the next environment is important, the most crucial factor in a successful transition to an inclusive environment for children with disabilities may be a positive working relationship between the family and the service providers (one study, focused on disability).

Conclusions from Family-Focused Studies

Two findings regarding families in transition were supported in the NECTC review by sufficient evidence to receive a rating of large evidence, using the *Extent of Evidence Categorization Scheme* (What Works Clearinghouse, 2008). A third finding met the first two criteria listed above, but not the third; that is, the total number of subjects in its seven supporting studies was 278, not 350 as predetermined for inclusion.

1. Transition is a complex process, not a static event. It is based on relationships. Positive relationships and transition support activities can ease the stress of transition for families (12 studies, most dealing with families of children with disabilities).
2. Parental sense of self-efficacy is associated with greater school-related parent involvement and improved academic outcomes for children (three studies, none focused on disability).
3. Needs of families must be met before families will be able to help their children with disabilities transition between programs or systems (seven studies, all including families of children with disabilities).

Thirteen studies reported families' agreement about the usefulness of transition support practices though these recommendations were not directly tested. The following practices were recommended by family members:

1. Provide families with options for future placements (five studies, all with families of children with disabilities).
2. Share information with families about their children's next environment, and give them ways to obtain answers to their questions about the new program (eight studies, including seven with families of children with disabilities).
3. Talk with families about accommodations and coping with expectations to help them reduce stress about their children's readiness for the next environment (four studies, including three with families of children with disabilities).
4. Provide transition planning and support tailored to meet the child's and family's needs (two studies, both with families of children with disabilities).
5. Work with interagency agreements and follow up to ensure a timely transfer of records, information about the child's special needs, and accommodations that will be necessary in the new environment (one study).
6. Provide families with contact information for individuals who can assist them with information and problem solving. Provide information in multiple formats and with redundancy to enable

them to assimilate the mass of complicated information (three studies, all with families of children with disabilities).

7. Involve families in all decisions regarding their children's future, including scheduling meetings at times and places that enable families to attend (three studies, all with families of children with disabilities).

8. Prepare the family to advocate for their child during transition and thereafter (two studies, both with families of children with disabilities).

9. Invite families to visit possible future environments and/or meet with the teacher (six studies, five with parents of children with disabilities).

10. Locate and refer families to community services that might supplement the program offered by special education (one study, with families of children with disabilities).

11. Include family participation on agency and interagency transition planning teams that develop the process and procedures (one study, with families of children with disabilities).

12. Link families of children with disabilities together through parent-to-parent activities and one-to-one mentoring (two studies, both with children with disabilities).

13. Provide follow-up support from the prekindergarten staff after the child has entered kindergarten via telephone calls, parent meetings, and additional information as requested (one study, with families of children with disabilities).

Conclusions from the NECTC Literature Search

According to the NECTC review (Rosenkoetter et al., 2008), while the focus on young children and their families in transition has been explored for at least 30 years, the current empirical research base for the transition of young children with disabilities is restricted in scope, focus, size, and rigor, and the results are fragmented. Further, studies of young children with disabilities and their families in transition have seldom been conducted in accord with conceptual models such as the ones presented here, lines of inquiry have been less than systematic, and specific transition practices have seldom been empirically linked to specific outcomes for children or families. The findings that were noted lend empirical support to the recommendations that the authors have observed in countless demonstration projects and technical assistance projects (Rosenkoetter, Whaley, Hains, & Pierce, 2001) and that have been widely publicized for 25 years, but additional investigation is needed to address the limitations cited.

NECTC National Validation Study

In much of the discussion about evidence-based practice, there has been agreement that both the scholarship of professionals and the experience of family members and service providers have relevance to key decisions about intervention (Buysse & Wesley, 2006). Honoring this principle, Rous (2008) set out to identify and validate a set of transition practices.

Twenty-one transition practices were identified from three studies (Rous, McCormick, & Hallam, 2006; Rous, Myers, & Stricklin, 2007; Rous, Schroeder, Stricklin, Hains, & Cox, 2008). A national survey was conducted with 419 early childhood and early childhood special education professionals to validate key practices that support the transition process as children leave early intervention and enter preschool and as they leave preschool and enter kindergarten. Of the 21 transition practices identified, all were validated by at least 75 percent of the respondents, while 20 were validated by 90 percent or more of the respondents (see Table 4.1). More information on the methods and findings of this study are available as Technical Report #3 at http://www.hdi.uky.edu/SF/NECTC/Publications/papers.aspx.

Table 4.1   Transition Practices Validated by NECTC

Interagency Service System (all approved by at least 90% of respondents)

1. A primary contact person for transition is identified within each program or agency.

2. Community- and program-wide transition activities and timelines are identified.

3. Referral processes and timelines are clearly specified.

4. Enrollment processes and timelines are clearly specified.

5. Program eligibility processes and timelines are clearly delineated.

6. Agencies develop formal mechanisms to minimize disruptions in services before, during, and after the transition of the child and family.

7. Staff and family members are actively involved in design of transition processes and systems.

(Continued)

Table 4.1 (Continued)

8. Staff roles and responsibilities for transition activities are clearly delineated.

9. Conscious and transparent connections are made between curricula and child expectations across programs/environments.

10. Methods are in place to support staff-to-staff communication within and across programs.

11. Families meaningfully participate as partners with staff in program- and community-wide transition efforts.

Child and Family Preparation and Adjustment (All except #2 were approved by at least 90% of respondents; it was approved by 75% of respondents)

1. Individual child and family transition meetings are conducted.

2. Staff follow up on children after the transition to support their adjustment.

3. Transition team members share appropriate information about each child making a transition.

4. Transition plans are developed that include individual activities for each child and family.

5. Staff know key information about a broad array of agencies and services available within the community.

6. Children have opportunities to develop and practice skills they need to be successful in the next environment.

7. Families are aware of the importance of transition planning and have information they need to actively participate in transition planning.

8. Families' needs related to transition are assessed and addressed.

9. Families have information about and are linked with resources and services to help them meet their specific child and family needs.

10. Families actively participate in gathering information about their child's growth and development.

Source: Rous (2008).

Findings from this multilevel approach provide empirical support for many of the guidelines that have been circulating for 25 years, and they validate the observations of parents, teachers, and administrators engaged in those practices. What continues to be lacking is linkage of the practices to specific outcomes of the transition process.

NECTC Critical Incident Study

Critical Incident Technique is a research strategy used to gather and analyze information from key informants about a significant experience in their lives (Flanagan, 1954). Transition from early intervention at age 3 or from preschool to kindergarten is such an experience for families and service providers of young children with disabilities (Rosenkoetter & Rosenkoetter, 2001). As reported by Dogaru, Rosenkoetter, and Rous (2009), NECTC sought comments nationwide from key informants representing these groups. Thirty-seven usable stories were recounted by parents of children with disabilities along with 28 by service providers.

Quotations from the respondents were found to address four themes: transition processes, evaluation of transition, transition outcomes, and family experiences in transition. Responses identified effective and ineffective practices, linked practices to child and family outcomes, and offered examples of salient events in transition. The study made clear that respectful communication, collaborative behaviors, timely actions, and family empowerment were judged to facilitate successful transition to a new environment by children with disabilities and their families.

Transition Research in Progress

Research on transition to kindergarten for children with disabilities and their families was declining in frequency prior to the USDOE's funding of the National Early Childhood Transition Center. It is anticipated that the release of findings from the Center's 18 studies will stimulate additional work by others. NECTC studies underway, in addition to those reported above, focus on young children with disabilities and include investigations of the kindergarten transition. Significant among them is a longitudinal, five-state study of 225 children at exit from early intervention, and 339 children at exit from preschool and their families, service providers/teachers, classrooms, programs, and states. Data are still under analysis, but the findings will help to answer these questions:

1. What are the characteristics of the transition process for children and families as they exit early intervention and preschool programs?
2. How do providers support the transition process for children and families as they exit from early intervention and preschool programs?
3. What are the characteristics of the transition process for children and families as they enter preschool and kindergarten programs?

4. How do preschool providers and providers support the transition process for children and families as they enter preschool and kindergarten programs?

The series of NECTC studies addresses both the contextual elements of the EDMT and NECTC models and the individual child and family elements. The findings also provide more clues, though not a full accounting of the relationships between transition practices and transition outcomes. Results will be aligned with the NECTC model, and the model itself may be modified pending the results of these investigations. Other NECTC research (see Harbin, Rous, Gooden, & Shaw, 2008) is exploring the state and community elements of transition to learn how structures, policies, recommended procedures and timelines, technical assistance, and resources link to transition outcomes. Those results will be forthcoming.

KEY PRINCIPLES FOR PRACTITIONERS

A successful transition "is influenced by the skills and behaviors the child exhibits during transition and the match between child skills and behaviors and the expectations and requirements of the receiving program" (Bruder & Chandler, 1996, p. 298). This comment sounds very much like the third definition of *school readiness* offered earlier in the chapter. Social, emotional, and academic adjustment to the new school's mores over a period of weeks is what makes the transition a successful or unsuccessful one for any child (Pianta & Kraft-Sayre, 1999), and the child's adjustment also determines how observers will ultimately evaluate the child's readiness for school. Though multiple systems certainly are instrumental in achieving a positive outcome, the focus of the transition to kindergarten continues to be at the child level.

Implications for Children

Although experiences vary by locale, by school, and even by teacher, most children will feel striking differences between prekindergarten and kindergarten. As noted above, the required adjustments may be greater for children with disabilities than for those without identified challenges (Carta & Atwater, 1990). Authors have defined these differences in three categories (Fowler et al., 1991; O'Brien, 1991; Rosenkoetter,

1995; Rosenkoetter, Hains, & Fowler, 1994; Rous & Hallam, 2006; Vail & Scott, 1994):

- *The environment:* This includes physical setting, building size and layout, classroom dimensions and arrangements, classroom equipment, adult/child ratio, length of sessions, daily schedule, and transportation plans; for example, most kindergarten classes are larger than prekindergarten classes, and many have only one teacher, unlike most prekindergarten classes.
- *Curriculum, expectations, and evaluations:* In kindergarten, the curriculum is typically more academic and structured, the materials more standardized, and the expectations more group oriented, evaluative, and regularly assessed than in prekindergarten.
- *Interactions and relationships with peers and teachers:* The role of the kindergarten teacher typically is to initiate activities, talk to the children frequently in a group, direct children's behavior, encourage their compliance, and organize activities for children, whereas in prekindergarten, activities are more likely to be child-directed for a significant portion of time once the teaching team has arranged the environment and provided choices of activities.

Interventions that are implemented to aid children in transition will promote self-care (Rule et al., 1990), membership in a group (Carta & Atwater, 1990), making friends (Peters, 2003), attention to task (McWilliam, Scarborough, & Kim, 2003), direction-following including introduction to the meaning of vocabulary used in schools (Rosenkoetter, 2001), and self-regulation (McClelland, Morrison, & Holmes, 2000). Interventions may reduce stress by visits prior to the beginning of the school year (Delisio, 2007), introduction to the classroom in small groups (Rosenkoetter, 2001), and direct teaching of the skills needed for kindergarten learning (Kemp & Carter, 2000; Rule et al., 1990: Sainato & Carta, 1992). These types of interventions focus on a within-the-child concept of school readiness.

However, in keeping with the Ready Schools notion of school readiness, school personnel also need to welcome the child who actually enters school and help the child feel welcome in what may feel like a very strange environment. Kindergarten personnel can support the child by learning about the child's special interests and needs, talking to prekindergarten personnel about effective intervention techniques, preparing in advance for accommodations noted in the Individualized

Education Program (IEP), mastering health and behavioral management techniques that may be needed, welcoming the parents, and planning ahead to aid the child's social integration (Rosenkoetter, Hains, & Fowler, 1994; SERVE, 1998; Wolery, 1999). Building a relationship of trust between the child and the teacher has been shown to affect eventual child achievement (O'Connor & McCartney, 2007).

Home visits have often been recommended by transition experts to allow kindergarten teachers to meet children and their families in their homes, hear their personal stories, answer questions, and build rapport. Schulting (2009a, 2009b) and Schulting and Dodge (2010) conducted a randomized, controlled trial of home visiting with 44 kindergarten teachers and approximately 928 families, including 81 percent minority and 28 percent non-English-speaking families. Interpretation was provided as needed. Home visits during the first five weeks of kindergarten led to statistically significant differences in child outcomes, teacher attitudes and beliefs, and parent involvement and communication over results obtained with teachers who did not conduct home visits. Effects were greatest for children from non-English-speaking homes. All participating kindergarten teachers said that they would conduct home visits every year if resources were available to enable them to occur. Nevertheless, only 4 percent of schools were found to conduct kindergarten home visits (Schulting, Malone, & Dodge, 2005), and the majority of teachers say that in their settings home visits are not practical (Pianta, Cox, Taylor, & Early, 1999).

Each of the transition practices to foster child and family adjustment that was validated by NECTC (see Table 4.1) supports the evidence-based approaches noted in the literature review as helping the kindergarten be ready for the child with disability that enrolls.

Implications for Families

The changes that families experience between prekindergarten and kindergarten may be significant. According to the findings of a study by Rimm-Kaufman and Pianta (1999), teacher-family contact occurs more frequently, is more informal, and is more positively oriented in prekindergarten than in kindergarten. The family-school relationship typically becomes more formal and less intense, as the new kindergarten setting usually offers fewer opportunities for parents to interact with school personnel.

In transition, parents of children with disabilities need to adjust to new schedules and routines for special education, attend IEP conferences with unfamiliar people in new places, and locate and access different technologies and services (Fowler et al., 1991). According to Harry (2002), Rosenkoetter and Rosenkoetter (2001), and Wolery (1999), the families of children with disabilities may face additional stressors, such as worrying how their children with disabilities will communicate their needs, how the children will fit into the new school environment, and how the unfamiliar teachers will treat their children. Some families show concern about discrimination and rejection of their children, the location and duration of their children's school day, the disability label to be applied perhaps for the first time, or the characteristics of school-provided transportation. Obviously, anything that the school can do to reduce these concerns will assist parents in supporting their children's kindergarten entry. Kemp (2003) noted how much the parents of children with disabilities whom she studied appreciated the supports provided to them by kindergarten personnel.

Pianta and Kraft-Sayre (1999) found that the criteria employed by parents of entering kindergartners for successful transition to kindergarten included (1) positive psychological responses by the child, (2) the development of parents' ongoing relationships with the school, (3) the impact of the prekindergarten on the child's adjustment to kindergarten, (4) families' effective communication with the school, (5) effective transition planning and transition activities, and (6) teacher and curriculum quality. For children with disabilities, Rosenkoetter and Rosenkoetter (2001) found parental concerns about transition were correlated with children's specific behavioral and emotional problems, such as concern that school expectations might be too high for children with limited cognition or worry about insufficient communication of needs for children with minimal language. Other specific concerns of parents for their children with disabilities were related to the child's riding a school bus, being safe on the playground, participating appropriately in large group activities, complying with rules and routines of the classroom, and following directions. Parental concerns increased with the severity of the child's disability, especially in the areas of self-care, ability to communicate the child's needs, and receipt of adequate services.

For all families, the transition to kindergarten has been found to be more successful when the parents become involved in their children's education as well as when they have higher self-esteem, increased confidence in the school and in themselves as parents, heightened expectations for their children, and greater social support (Henderson & Berla, 1994). According to these research findings, the transition to kindergarten is more successful when parents are empowered to work with their children's learning and to participate at school as well as when they become more skilled in the four parental roles that promote their children's success in school: teacher, supporter, advocate, and decision maker. The list of transition practices to foster child and family adjustment that was validated by NECTC (see Table 4.1) support the approaches emphasized from the literature review to help the kindergarten be ready for the family of the child with disability.

Implications for Service Providers

Obviously, individual child and family characteristics influence the nature of the transition to kindergarten (Kemp, 2003), but, notably, its success depends on comprehensive collaboration, ongoing co-operation, and timely and respectful communication among the parties involved (Athanasiou, 2006; Bruder & Chandler, 1996; Fowler et al., 1991; Mangione & Speth, 1998). Clearly, the delivery of such coordinated transition services by personnel from multiple systems requires transition planning (Rosenkoetter, Hains, & Fowler, 1994; Rous & Hallam, 2006; Wolery, 1999). The purposes of this planning by representatives of the multiple systems are, in the words of the NECTC model, (1) alignment and continuity, (2) supportive infrastructure, and (3) communication and relationships. The transition practices to foster child and family adjustment that were validated by NECTC (see Table 4.1) provide empirical support to guide service providers' actions.

Transition: Why Is It So Difficult?

Federal, state, and local agencies and numerous individuals have worked since at least the 1970s to ease early childhood transitions. Countless families have expended considerable efforts in trying to make transition "work" for their children. Most participants approach transition with good will, good intentions, and the commitment of time and energy. In the majority of cases, children adjust and learn, and families participate in the transition and advocate for their children, but enough difficulties remain that thoughtful observers continue to seek to understand and alleviate the challenges.

As described above in the discussion of models, transition to kindergarten represents a supra-system made up of component systems, which, in turn, contain subsystems. These various participants in the process represent different interests, hold different powers in decision making, and experience diverse events related to one child's entry into kindergarten. Personnel and their agencies view the transition from different vantage points. Using the concepts of Bolman and Deal (2008), we see four frames or lenses (and combinations of them) through which various transition participants may view transition:

- *The structural frame:* This lens is exemplified by flow charts, timelines, organization charts, memoranda of understanding, precedents, laws, and regulations. These elements are the important and necessary tools of the midlevel planners who understand early childhood practice and grasp the big picture of the transition process for groups of children, more consistently, perhaps, than they see the individual characteristics of day-to-day transition participants. These leaders may also be challenged to communicate with spokespersons from supra-systems, who may not understand the philosophy and issues of work with young children.

- *The human resources frame:* This viewpoint is exemplified by relationship building, degrees of respect, personality matching, trust, and satisfaction of needs. These transition elements are the priorities of transition participants such as family members and direct service providers who focus attention on the needs, preferences, and talents of individual children and their families.

- *The political frame:* This viewpoint is exemplified by policy, power, budgets, negotiation, scarce resources, and leverage. These elements are critical in delivering services. They are the special province of administrators, who typically assess their own clout and that of their agency in collaborative endeavors and then use the resources that they have available to move transition decisions forward.

- *The symbolic frame:* This lens is exemplified by concepts such as milestone, beginning of school career, family partnership, collaborative decision making, and moving forward together. Truly, transition to kindergarten is a big step for everyone involved. It symbolizes the commitment of the school to the child and family, of the child to a lifetime of learning, and of the family to support their child in an important new experience. Some symbols are discussed in transition interactions, but others are not because they may be below the level of awareness of most transition participants.

Each of these four frames, plus their accompanying responsibilities and tasks, has an important role to play in transition planning. To make transition work, participants must understand their own frames as well as those of the other participants, and they must develop ways to satisfy the needs of participants with different points of view and varying constraints. At the same time, they must focus on easing the transition to kindergarten for the child with a disability and the child's family. Nearly every participant has blind spots related to the transition process as well as competing pressures for time and attention. Unfortunately, as the transition-planning process moves forward, personnel may change, resulting in the need for transition planners to revisit familiar ground, listen, learn, and negotiate procedures and decisions yet again. Written memoranda of understanding can help to alleviate blind spots and gaps in responsibility (Fink, Borgia, & Fowler, 1993). Shared purpose, frequently articulated, is the avenue for progress in transition planning.

Bruder and Chandler (1996) stated that transition efforts should be comprehensive and should address multiple components, including formal planning, implementation, and follow-up. Yet many communities appear to have limited plans in place, or plans that have not been reaffirmed with the current transition leaders. Revisiting the Bolman and Deal (2008) framework along with one of the models presented above may help community planners to move forward to achieve consistently positive outcomes for children and families.

FUTURE DIRECTIONS FOR TRANSITION RESEARCH

The most striking finding from the review conducted by NECTC on child and family issues at transition was the paucity of data-based, peer-reviewed studies. Further, most existing studies related to disability were descriptive in nature. NECTC and others (e.g., Connelly, 2007) are enhancing the research base. A key recommendation for the research community is to fund and conduct more research, especially studies that test strategies to facilitate transition to kindergarten and those that link the use of particular transition practices for children with disabilities and/or their family members with meaningful outcomes that have been shown to have long-term impact. The first step, validation of promoted transition practices, has now been accomplished by several studies. Work has begun on correlations between initial contextual and child-readiness characteristics and subsequent child adjustment to and performance in school (e.g., Greenberg, Lengua, Coie, & Pinderhughes, 1999; Miller et al., 2003; Mistry, Biesanz, Taylor, Burchinal, & Cox, 2004; Silver, Measelle, Armstrong, & Essex, 2004) as well as on correlations between various transition characteristics and subsequent child performance and family engagement (Schulting, Malone, & Dodge, 2005). It remains for research to demonstrate more clearly the long-term behavioral impact of transition practices on child and family outcomes. Causality and its mechanisms are the missing demonstrations that will challenge the next generation of transition researchers.

Critical to achieving a worthy research agenda for the next decade is for researchers to build their inquiry on a conceptual framework such as that proposed by NECTC, a model that incorporates contexts, dynamic elements hypothesized or demonstrated to be critical for positive change, practices and strategies proposed for intervention, and child and family outcomes, both short term and long term. Launching inquiries from a conceptual framework will foster clarity in thinking. It will help to identify which notions already possess clear evidence, highlight gaps in knowledge, promote the study of pivotal interactions, and help scholars to focus on key questions. Use of a conceptual framework will promote the replication of existing research with various populations, including those that have been inadequately studied to date. Populations where transition research has only recently begun and that present challenging issues for practice include children and families from underrepresented racial, ethnic, and cultural groups; individuals whose first language is not standard English; children with significant disabilities; and family members who themselves evidence disability.

Other obvious questions involve empirical evidence for discrete transition practices, the relative importance of various practices, a cost-benefit analysis of specific approaches, and the identification of focal children and families who can most benefit from particular practices. For example, it became obvious during interviews connected with the NECTC longitudinal study that a child with a communication disability would likely need different accommodations and different family support during transition to kindergarten than a child with severe cerebral palsy or a major medical condition. Similarly, a family new to the special education system, the health care system, or the community's social service system, or one suddenly aware of the need for family advocacy, might require different kinds of transition support than a family that has been involved in all of the above since their child's infancy. Rosenkoetter and Rosenkoetter (2001) found that parents whose oldest or only child was entering kindergarten had many more questions and concerns than those who had successfully navigated this same transition with older children. Sontag and Schacht (1994) found different information needs among parents of various ethnicities in early intervention. Use of a conceptual framework will likely increase the number, quality, and precision of research questions that extend the evidence for specific transition practices.

Finally, more research findings on transition for young children with disability are now becoming available. Its findings need to be conveyed in formats that can be easily digested and applied by parents and professionals who are not experts in this area. Family members, physicians, social workers, educators, psychologists, administrators, and therapists of various types need concise, clear, specific guidance as to how to ease transition to kindergarten for young children with disabilities and their families. Limited national and state efforts are underway to make such guidance accessible. Further efforts along these lines should be encouraged, with awareness of the various frames that consumers of information bring to their understanding of transition.

REFERENCES

Athanasiou, M. S. (2006). It takes a village: Children's transition to kindergarten. *School Psychology Quarterly, 21*(4), 468–473.

Bolman, L. G., & Deal, T. E. (2008). *Reframing organizations: Artistry, choice, and leadership.* San Francisco: Jossey-Bass.

Bruder, M. B., & Chandler, L. (1996). Transition. In S. L. Odom & M. E. McLean (Eds.), *Early intervention/early childhood special education: Recommended practices* (pp. 287–307). Austin, TX: PRO-ED.

Buysse, V., & Wesley, P. W. (2006). *Evidence-based practice in the early childhood field.* Washington, DC: Zero to Three Press.

Carta, J. J., & Atwater, J. B. (1990). Applications of ecobehavioral analysis to the study of transitions across early education settings. *Education and Treatment of Children, 13,* 4298–4315.

Connelly, A. M. (2007). Transitions of families from early intervention to preschool intervention for children with disabilities. *Young Exceptional Children, 10*(3), 10–16.

Delisio, E. R. (2007). Rounding up pre-k kids. *Education World.* Retrieved from http://www.education-world.com/a_admin/admin/admin359.shtml

Deming, D., & Dynarski, S. (2008). The lengthening of childhood. *Journal of Economic Perspectives, 22*(3), 71–92.

Dogaru, C. M. (2008). *Applying theories of capital to understand parent involvement at school as a component of family-school interaction: The special case of children with special needs* (doctoral dissertation submitted to Oregon State University).

Dogaru, C., Rosenkoetter, S., & Rous, B. (2009). *A critical incident study of the transition experience for young children with disabilities: Recounts by parents and professionals: Technical Report #6.* Lexington: University of Kentucky, Human Development Institute. National Early Childhood Transition Center. Available at http://www.hdi.uky.edu/SF/NECTC/Publications/papers.aspx

Eccles, J. S., & Harold, R. D. (1996). Family involvement in children's and adolescents' schooling. In A. Booth & F. Dunn (Eds.), *Family-school links. How do they affect educational outcomes?* (pp. 3–34). Mahwah, NJ: Lawrence Erlbaum Associates, Inc.

Education Week. (2004, September 21). English-language learners. Retrieved from http://www.edweek.org/rc/issues/english-language-learners

Fink, D., Borgia, E., & Fowler, S. A. (Ed.). (1993). *Interagency agreements: Improving the transition process for young children with special needs and their families.* Champaign-Urbana: University of Illinois, FACTS/LRE.

Flanagan, J. C. (1954). The Critical incident technique. *Psychological Bulletin, 51*(4), 327–358.

Ford, D. H., & Lerner, R. M. (1992). *Developmental systems theory: An integrative approach.* Thousand Oaks, CA: Sage Publications.

Fowler, S. A. (1982). Transition from preschool to kindergarten for children with special needs. In K. E. Allen and E. M. Goetz (Eds.) *Early childhood education: Special problems, special solutions* (pp. 229–242). Rockville, MD: Aspen.

Fowler, S. A., Schwartz, I., & Atwater, J. (1991). Perspectives on the transition from preschool to kindergarten for children with disabilities and their families. *Exceptional Children, 58*(2), 136–145.

Frey, N. (2005). Retention, social promotion, and academic redshirting: What do we know? *Remedial and Special Education, 26,* 332–346.

Graue, M. E. (1993). *Ready for what? Constructing meanings of readiness for kindergarten.* Albany: State University of New York Press.

Gredler, G. (2006). Transition classes: A viable alternative for the at-risk child. *Psychology in the Schools, 21*(4), 463–470.

Greenberg, M. T., Lengua, L. J., Coie, J. D., & Pinderhughes, E. E. (1999). Predicting developmental outcomes at school entry using a multiple-risk model: Four American communities. *Developmental Psychology, 35,* 403–417.

Harbin, G., Rous, B., Gooden, C., & Shaw, J. (2008). *State infrastructures to support young children with disabilities: Technical report #4.* Lexington: University of Kentucky, Human Development Institute. Available at http://www.hdi.uky.edu/SF/NECTC/Publications/papers.aspx

Harbin, G., Rous, B., & McLean, M. (2004). *Issues in designing state accountability systems.* Chapel Hill, NC: Frank Porter Graham Child Development Center.

Harbin, G., Rous, B., Peeler, N., Schuster, J., & McCormick, K. (December, 2007). *Desired family outcomes of the early childhood transition process: Research brief.* Lexington: University of Kentucky, Human Development Institute. Retrieved from http://www.hdi.uky.edu/SF/NECTC/Publications/resbriefs.aspx

Harry, B. (2002). Trends and issues in serving culturally diverse families of children with disabilities. *Journal of Special Education, 36,* 131–138.

Head Start Act of 2003. U.S. Code, 42USC 9801. Public Law 105-285, Section 641A. Title 45, Chapter XIII, Part. 1304.

Head Start Bureau. (1989). *Transition.* Washington, DC: Administration for Children, Youth, and Families.

Head Start Child Outcomes Framework. (n.d.) Retrieved from http://www.hsnrc.org/CDI/pdfs/UGCOF.pdf

Hebbeler, K., & Barton, L. (2007). The need for data on child and family outcomes at the Federal and State levels. *Young Exceptional Children Monograph Series, 9,* 1–15.

Hebbeler, K., Barton, L. R., & Mallik, S. (2008). Assessment and accountability for programs serving young children with disabilities. *Exceptionality, 16*(1), 48–63.

Henderson, A. T., & Berla, N. (1994). *A new generation of evidence: The family is critical to student achievement.* Washington, DC: Center of Law and Education.

Hoover-Dempsey, K. V., & Sandler, H. M. (1997). Parental involvement in children's education: why does it make a difference? *Teachers College Record, 97*(2), 310–332.

Ilg, F., Ames, L., Haines, J., & Gillespie, C. (1978). *School readiness: Behavior tests used at the Gesell Institute.* New York: Harper & Row.

Individuals with Disabilities Education Improvement Act of 2004. Public Law, No. 1 108-466 & 632, 118 State. 2744.

Kagan, S. L., Moore, E., & Bredekamp, S. (Eds.). (1995). *Reconsidering children's early development and learning: Toward shared beliefs and vocabulary.* Washington, DC: National Education Goals Panel.

Katims, D. S., & Pierce, P. L. (1995). Literary-rich environments and the transition of young children with special needs. *Topics in Early Childhood Special Education, 15*(2), 219–234.

Kemp, C. (2003). Investigating the transition of young children with intellectual disabilities to mainstream classes: An Australian perspective. *International Journal of Disability, Development, and Education, 50,* 403–433.

Kemp, C., & Carter, M. (2000). Demonstration of classroom survival skills in kindergarten: A five-year transition study of children with intellectual disabilities. *Educational Psychology, 20*(4), 393–411.

Ladd, G. (2006). Peer rejections, aggressive or withdrawn behavior, and psychological maladjustment from ages 5 to 12: An examination of four predictive models. *Child Development.*

Lazzari. A. M. (1991). *The transition sourcebook: A practical guide for early intervention programs.* Tucson, AZ: Communication Skill Builders.

Love, J. M., Logue, M. E., Trudeau, J. V., & Thayer, K. (1992). *Transitions to kindergarten in American schools.* Hampton, NH: RCM Research Corporation.

Mangione, P. L., & Speth, T. (1998). The transition to elementary school: A framework for creating early childhood continuity through home, school, and community partnership. *Elementary School Journal, 98*(4), 381–397.

Mantzicopoulos, P. (2003). Academic and school adjustment outcomes following placement in a developmental first-grade program. *Journal of Educational Research, 97*(2), 90–105.

McClelland, M. M., Morrison, F. J., & Holmes, D. L. (2000). Children at-risk for early academic problems: The role of learning-related social skills. *Early Childhood Research Quarterly, 15,* 307–329.

McWilliam, R. A., Scarborough, A. A., & Kim, H. (2003). Adult interactions and child engagement. *Early Education and Development, 14,* 7–27.

Miller, A., Gouley, K. K., Shields, A., Dickstein, S., Seifer, R., Dodge-Magee, K., et al. (2003). Brief functional screening for transition difficulties prior to enrollment predicts socio-emotional competence and school adjustment in Head Start preschoolers. *Early Child Development and Care, 173,* 681–698.

Mistry, R. S., Biesanz, J. C., Taylor, L. C., Burchinal, M., & Cox, M. J. (2004). Family income and its relation to preschool children's adjustment for families in the NICHD study of early child care. *Developmental Psychology, 40,* 727–745.

National Association for the Education of Young Children. (1990).NAEYC position statement on school readiness. *Young Children, 46*(1), 21–23.

National Association for the Education of Young Children. (1995). *School readiness: A position statement of the NAEYC.* Retrieved from http://www.naeyc.org/positionstatements

National Center for Education Statistics. (2009). *Characteristics of children in early childhood programs: Fast facts.* Washington, DC: U.S. Department of Education. Retrieved from http://nces.ed.gov/fastfacts

National Early Childhood Accountability Task Force, T. Schultz, & S. L. Kagan (Eds). (2007). *Taking stock: Assessing and improving early childhood learning and program quality.* Washington, DC: Pew Charitable Trusts.

National Education Goals Panel, Goal 1: Ready Schools Resource Group (R. Shore, Ed.). (1998). *Ready schools.* Washington, DC: Author. Retrieved from http://govinfo.library.unt.edu/negp/reports/readysch

National Education Goals Panel, Goal 1: Technical Planning Group (S. L. Kagan, E. Moore, & S. Bredekamp, Eds.) (1995). *Reconsidering children's early development and learning: Toward common views and vocabulary.* Washington, DC: Author.

No Child Left Behind Act of 2001. Public Law 107-87, Statutue 1425, enacted January 8, 2002.

O'Brien, M. (1991). *Promoting successful transition into school: A review of current intervention practices.* Lawrence: Kansas Early Childhood Research Institute.

O'Connor, E., & McCartney, K. (2007). Examining teacher-child relationships and achievement as part of an ecological model of development. *American Educational Research Journal, 44*(2), 340–369.

Peters, S. (2003). "I didn't expect that I would get tons of friends . . . more each day": Children's experiences of friendship during the transition to school. *Early Years: An International Journal of Research and Development, 23,* 45–53.

Pianta, R. C., & Cox, M. J. (1999). *The transition to kindergarten.* Baltimore: Paul H. Brookes.

Pianta, R. C., Cox, M. J., Taylor, L., & Early, D. (1999). Kindergarten teachers' practices related to transition to school: Results of a national survey. *The Elementary School Journal, 100*(1), 71–86.

Pianta, R. C., & Kraft-Sayre, M. (1999). Parents' observations about their children's transitions to kindergarten. *Young Children, 54,* 47–52.

Pianta, R. C., & Kraft-Sayre, M. (2003). *Successful kindergarten transition: Your guide to connecting children, families, and schools.* Baltimore: Paul H. Brookes.

Pianta, R. C., & Walsh, D. J. (1996). *High risk children in the schools: Creating sustaining relationships.* New York: Routledge.

Ramey, S. L., & Ramey, C. T. (1994). The transition to school: Why the first few years matter for a lifetime. *Phi Delta Kappan, 76,* 3194–3198.

Ramey, C. T., & Ramey, S. L. (1998). Commentary: The transition to school: Opportunities for children, families, educators and communities. *Elementary School Journal, 98*(4), 293–295.

Rimm-Kaufman, S. E., & Pianta, R. C. (1999). Patterns of family-school contact in preschool and kindergarten. *School Psychology Review, 28*(3), 426–438.

Rimm-Kaufman, S. E., & Pianta, R. C. (2000). An ecological perspective on the transition to kindergarten: A theoretical framework to guide transition. *Journal of Applied Developmental Psychology, 21*(5), 491–511.

Rist, R. (1970). Student social class and teacher expectations: The self-fulfilling prophecy in ghetto education. *Harvard Educational Review, 40*(3), 411–451.

Rosenkoetter, S. E. (Ed.). (1995). *It's a big step.* Topeka, KS: Bridging Early Services Transition Taskforce.

Rosenkoetter, S. E. (2001). Lessons for preschool language socialization from the vantage point of the first day of kindergarten. *Early Education and Development, 12*(3), 325–342.

Rosenkoetter, S. E., Hains, A. H., & Fowler, S. A. (1994). *Bridging early services for children with special needs and their families: A practical guide for transition planning.* Baltimore: Paul H. Brookes.

Rosenkoetter, S. E., & Rosenkoetter, L. I. (2001). Starting school: Parents' perceptions regarding their typically developing children and those with disabilities. *Dialog: The Research Journal of the National Head Start Association, 4*(2), 223–245.

Rosenkoetter, S, Schroeder, C., Hains, A., Rous, B., & Shaw, J. (2008). *A review of research in early childhood transition: Child and family studies: Technical report #5.* Lexington: University of Kentucky, Human Development Institute, National Early Childhood Transition Center. Available at http://www.hdi.uky.edu/SF/NECTC/Publications/papers.aspx

Rosenkoetter, S. E., Whaley, K. T., Hains, A. T., & Pierce, L. (2001). The evolution of transition policy for young children with special needs and their families: Past, present, and future. *Topics in Early Childhood Special Education, 21*(1), 3–15.

Rous, B. (2008). *Recommended transition practices for young children and families: National validation survey: Technical Report #3.* Lexington: University of Kentucky, Human Development Institute. National Early Childhood Transition Center. Available at http://www.hdi.uky.edu/SF/NECTC/Publications/papers.aspx

Rous, B. S., & Hallam, R. A. (2006). *Tools for transition in early childhood: A step-by step guide for agencies, teachers, and families.* Baltimore: Paul H. Brookes.

Rous, B., Hallam, R., Harbin, G. McCormick, K., & Jung, L. A. (2007). The transition process for young children with disabilities: A conceptual framework. *Infants and Young Children, 20*(2), 135–148.

Rous, B., LoBianco, T., Moffett, C. L., & Lund, I. (2005). Building preschool accountability systems: Guidelines resulting from a national study. *Journal of Early Intervention, 28*(1).

Rous, B., McCormick, K., & Hallam, R. (2006). *Use of transition practices by public school teachers: Research brief.* Lexington: University of Kentucky, Human Development Institute, National Early Childhood Transition Center. Available at http://www.hdi.uky.edu/SF/NECTC/Publications/resbriefs.aspx

Rous, B., Myers, C. T., & Stricklin, S. (2007). Strategies for supporting transitions for young children with special needs. *Journal of Early Intervention, 30*(1), 1–18.

Rous, B., Schroeder, C., Stricklin, S. G., Hains, A., & Cox, M. (2008). *Transition issues and barriers for children with significant disabilities and from culturally and linguistically diverse backgrounds: Technical report #2.* Lexington: University of Kentucky, Human Development Institute, National Early Childhood Transition Center.

Rule, S., Feichtl, B. J., & Innocenti, M. S. (1990). Preparation for transition to main-streamed post-preschool environments: Development of a survival skills curriculum. *Topics in Early Childhood Special Education, 9*, 78–90.

Sainato, D. M., & Carta, J. J. (1992). Classroom influences on the development of social competence of preschool children with disabilities: Ecology, teachers, and peers. In S. L. Odom, S. R. McConnell, & M. A. McEvoy (Eds.) *Social competence of young children with disabilities: Issues and strategies for intervention*. Baltimore: Paul H. Brookes.

Schulting, A. (2009a). *The kindergarten home visit project: Enhancing the transition to kindergarten*. Durham, NC: Duke University, Center for Child and Family Policy. Retrieved from http://childandfamilypolicy.duke.edu/pdfs/schoolresearch/SRP_Kindergarten_visit_2009.pps

Schulting, A. (2009b). The kindergarten home visit project. Retrieved from http://www.hfrp.org/family-involvement/publications-resources/kindergarten-home-visit-project

Schulting, A. B., & Dodge, K. A. (2010). The kindergarten home visit project: A kindergarten transition intervention study. Manuscript under editorial review. Durham, NC: Duke University.

Schulting, A. B., Malone, P. S., & Dodge, K. A. (2005). The effect of school-based kindergarten transition policies and practices on child academic outcomes. *Developmental Psychology, 41*, 860–871.

Scott-Little, C., Kagan, S. L., & Frelow, V. S. (2005). Inside the content: The breadth and depth of early learning standards. *Creating the conditions for success with early learning standards*. Greensboro, NC: University of North Carolina.

Scott-Little, C., Kagan, S. L., Frelow, V. S., & Reid, J. (2008). *Inside the content of infant-toddler early learning guidelines: Results from analyses, issues to consider, and recommendations*. Greensboro, NC: University of North Carolina at Greensboro.

SERVE. (1998). *Terrific transitions: Ensuring continuity of services for children and their families*. Greensboro, NC: Southeastern Regional Vision for Education.

Silver, R. B., Measelle, J. R., Armstrong, J. M., & Essex, M. J. (2004). Trajectories of classroom externalizing behavior: Contributions of child characteristics, family characteristics, and the teacher-child relationship during the school transition. *Journal of School Psychology, 43*, 39–60.

Smith, E. P., Connel, C. M., Wright, G., Sizer, M., & Norman, J. M. (1997). An ecological model of home, school, and community partnership: Implications for research and practice. *Journal of Educational and Psychological Consultation, 8*(4), 339–360.

Sontag, J. C., & Schacht, R. (1994). An ethnic comparison of parent participation and information needs in early intervention. *Exceptional Children, 60*(5), 422–433.

Stipek, D. (2002). At what age should children enter kindergarten? A question for policy makers and parents. *Social Policy Report, 16*(2), 3–17. Retrieved from http://www.srcd.org/index.php?option=com_docman&task=doc_download&gid=120

Task Force on School Readiness. (2005). *Building the foundation for bright futures: Final report of the NGA Task Force on School Readiness*. Washington, DC: National Governors' Association.

Turnbull, A., Turnbull, R., & Wehmeyer, M. L. (2007). *Exceptional lives: Special education in today's schools*. Upper Saddle River, NJ: Pearson/Merrill/Prentice Hall.

U.S. Department of Education. (1991). *Preparing young children for success: Guideposts for achieving our first national education goal*. Washington, DC: Author.

U.S. Department of Education. (2009). *Dropout rates: Fast facts*. Retrieved from http://nces.ed.gov/fastfacts

U.S. Department of Education, Office of Special Education and Rehabilitation. (2006). *28th annual report to Congress on the implementation the Individuals with Disabilities Education Act* (Vol. 1). Washington, DC: Author. Retrieved from http://www.ed.gov/about/reports/annual/osep/2006

Vail, C. O., & Scott, K. S. (1994). Transition from preschool to kindergarten for children with special needs: Issues for early childhood education. *Dimensions of Early Childhood, 22*(3), 21–25.

What Works Clearinghouse. (2008). *WWC procedures and standards handbook: Extent of evidence categorization scheme*. Princeton, NJ: U.S. Department of Education, Institute of Education Sciences, National Center for Educational Evaluation and Regional Assistance, What Works Clearinghouse.

Wolery, M. (1999). Children with disabilities in early elementary school. In R. C. Pianta & M. J. Cox (Eds.), *The transition to kindergarten* (pp. 253–280). Baltimore: Paul H. Brookes.

Zill, N. (1999). Promoting educational equity and excellence in kindergarten. In R. C. Pianta & M. J. Cox (Eds.), *The transition to kindergarten* (pp. 67–105). Baltimore: Paul H. Brookes.

Chapter 5

Uses of Technology in Early Intervention

Amy G. Dell, Deborah A. Newton, and Jerry G. Petroff

Assistive technology can provide a voice for children who cannot speak (Arnold, 2003; Fried-Oken & Bersani, 2000; Williams, 2006). It can provide access to mobility (i.e., power wheelchairs) for children who cannot walk. It offers opportunities for young children to play even if they cannot manipulate toys or art materials (Mistrett et al., 2006). Technology can enable young children to participate in daily routines that take place in every home and preschool. It can enable young children to demonstrate their understanding of cognitive concepts even if their disabilities prevent them from performing on standard assessments (Male, 2003). Technology can provide access to the general early childhood curriculum and key educational experiences such as early literacy. Access to the curriculum is a critical component of the successful inclusion of children with disabilities in their neighborhood schools (Nolet & McLaughlin, 2000; Salend, 2004; Villa & Thousand, 2000). Appropriate uses of technology can decrease children's reliance on teachers and parents by increasing their independence in many activities (Bryant, Bryant, & Rieth, 2002).

However, technology by itself is useless. Providing young children who have disabilities with the latest, most dazzling devices in the world will not make a difference in their lives unless the initiative integrates the technology into the child's curriculum, addresses the details of implementation, and makes sure everyone involved receives appropriate training (Burkhart, n.d.). Therefore, this chapter's emphasis is on the integration of assistive technology into the early intervention curriculum—how assistive technology can be used in all kinds of environments to enhance the teaching and learning of young children with a wide range of disabilities (PACER Center, 2006). Although it is easy to be seduced by the razzle-dazzle of the latest electronic gizmo, it is important to resist that temptation and instead focus on the *link* between technology and the teaching-learning process. The context for our discussion of technology in early intervention is always the environments and activities in which young children participate and learn. This approach reflects the philosophy of the leading professional organization in educational technology, the International Society for Technology in Education (ISTE), which articulates that "learning with technology should not be about the technology itself but about the learning that can be facilitated through it" (Knezek, Christensen, Bell, & Bull, 2006, p. 19).

WHAT IS ASSISTIVE TECHNOLOGY?

The important role assistive technology can play in the education of children with disabilities is underscored by its inclusion in the most recent reauthorization of the Individuals with Disabilities Education Act (IDEA, 2004). IDEA defines the term "assistive technology" by breaking it down into two parts: assistive technology *devices*, and assistive technology *services*. The delineating of both components is extremely important.

IDEA 2004 defines an assistive technology *device* as "any item, piece of equipment, or product system, whether acquired commercially off the shelf, modified, or customized, that is used to increase, maintain, or improve functional capabilities of a child with a disability" (IDEA 2004, Sec. 1401[1][A]). Let us examine this definition in reverse. An assistive technology device must have an impact on the *functioning* of a child with a disability. For example, a portable magnifier enables a child who has a visual impairment to see the pictures and words in a picture book, thereby improving the child's ability to develop literacy. A motorized wheelchair increases the ability of a child who has a physical disability to move around his or her environment to interact with other children and participate in play activities. A talking augmentative communication system for a child with autism increases the child's ability to communicate and enables him or her to make choices. These three examples show how an assistive technology device can "increase, maintain, or improve functional capabilities of a child with a disability."

The first part of the definition tells us that an assistive technology device can be bought in a store ("acquired commercially off the shelf"), it can be a purchased item that has been "modified," or it can be something that has been customized for a child's particular needs. A large computer monitor is an example of an assistive technology device that can be bought in a store (for children with visual impairments who need an enlarged visual display). Another example of "off the shelf" assistive technology is a talking picture book that uses sound chips to read aloud the text and provide sound effects, both of which engage children with attention problems.

Examples of modifications to "off the shelf products" include adding wooden blocks to the pedals of a tricycle so a child who has short legs can reach the pedals; building up the handle of an eating utensil with foam so a child with poor motor skills can grip and manipulate it better; and adding special software to a standard computer so a child with developmental delays can learn pre-academic skills.

Customized assistive technology devices include a wide variety of items. Communication boards created with pictures and talking computerized devices that serve as augmentative communication devices are usually customized for each individual child. Teacher-made computer-based activities for the teaching of specific skills are another example of customized assistive technology devices.

Assistive Technology Continuum

As you can see from these examples, the definition of assistive technology devices is quite broad. A helpful way of organizing all of these possibilities is to place them on an assistive technology continuum—that is, a continuum from "low-tech" to "high-tech." Low-tech devices use no electronic components and are relatively inexpensive. They are what are often called "gadgets," "gizmos," "doodads," or "thingamajigs," that is, "simple tools that make life's daily activities easier" (Collins, n.d.). A cookbook stand that holds open the pages of a cookbook so a cook can refer to it easily makes a terrific low-tech book holder for a preschooler whose cerebral palsy prevents him from holding a book independently. Oversized crayons, markers, and paint brushes; "chubby" paint rollers; and pencil grips that build up the shaft of a pencil to improve a child's control are examples of low-tech aids for coloring, drawing, painting, and writing, as are clipboards that can be used to hold sheets of paper steady.

"High-tech" devices are items that often are based on computer technology. In general, high-tech devices are more complicated to operate than low-tech devices, require more training than low-tech devices, and are considerably more expensive. However, high-tech devices offer unique benefits that often make their expense and training demands worthwhile. They are powerful and flexible devices, and can be used for many different tasks. For example, desktop computers and laptop computers connected to the Internet and equipped with specialized software can be used for early writing, reading, and learning new skills. Sophisticated augmentative communication systems can be used to provide a voice for children who cannot speak.

In between sophisticated high-tech devices and non-electronic low-tech devices are items classified as "mid-tech" devices. Mid-tech devices are electronic in nature but are much less expensive and require less training than high-tech devices. Digital recorders for recording stories and CD players for reading stories aloud are examples of mid-tech devices. Low-end augmentative communication devices, such as the Go-Talk (Attainment), are other examples of mid-tech devices.

IDEA's definition of assistive technology includes an exception—"The term 'assistive technology device' does *not* include a medical device that is surgically implanted, or the replacement of such device" (IDEA, 2004, Sec. 1401[1][B]). For example, feeding tubes for children who cannot eat and cochlear implants for children who are deaf represent implanted devices that are not considered assistive technology under IDEA.

Assistive Technology Services

The second part of IDEA's definition of assistive technology addresses assistive technology *services*. The term "assistive technology service" refers to "any service that directly assists a child with a disability in the selection, acquisition, or use of an assistive technology device" (IDEA, 2004, Sec. 1401[2]). Assistive technology services include evaluating a child for assistive technology, purchasing or leasing an assistive technology device for a child, customizing a device to meet a child's specific needs, repairing or replacing a broken device, teaching the child to use the device, and providing training for professionals who work with the child and/or for family members who are "substantially involved in the major life functions" of the child (IDEA, 2004, Sec. 1401[2][F]). The inclusion of assistive technology services in the law is extremely important as it recognizes that simply *providing* a device is not enough. The law's wording is public acknowledgement that making a device available without providing essential supports will not lead to successful implementation of assistive technology.

ASSISTIVE TECHNOLOGY DECISION MAKING

IDEA mandates that assistive technology be considered for every child receiving services under the law, including infants and toddlers under Part C. A young child should be considered a candidate for an assistive technology device and service(s) when the child is unable to perform activities that typical peers engage in, and the inability to display these skills is having a negative impact on the child's participation in activities and routines (Pennsylvania Training and Technical Assistance Network, 2005).

Determining *which* assistive technology tools will benefit a child is a critical first step. This process is referred to as assistive technology assessment, or assistive technology decision making. The literature on best practices is very clear on the characteristics of exemplary assistive technology assessments. Decisions about assistive technology must include the following six elements (QIAT Consortium, 2005):

1. Use of a team approach
2. Focus on student needs and abilities
3. Examination of tasks to be completed
4. Consideration of relevant environmental issues
5. Provision of necessary supports
6. Use of assessment information

Use of a team approach: Decisions about assistive technology selection should never be made by one person working alone. Teachers, parents, occupational therapists, physical therapists, speech language pathologists, and others all have in-depth knowledge but possibly different perspectives on a particular child. They, along with assistive technology specialists, have a wealth of assistive technology information and expertise as it relates to their individual fields. Working together, they are more likely to meet a student's assistive technology needs than any one of them working in isolation.

Focus on the child's needs and abilities: Assistive technology assessments must always be child-centered, identifying technology tools that will meet a child's individual needs; the available technology should never drive the assessment process. Although it is easy to be captivated by the latest gizmos and accompanying media hype, teams must start the process with the child, and must match the technology to the child (QIAT Consortium, 2005; Zabala, 2009).

Examination of tasks to be completed: In addition to knowing about the child's needs and abilities, the team needs to answer the question, in which activities does the child's participation and/or independence need to increase? In which part of the activity does the child need support? For example, is the child's play limited to passive observing of other children? Does the child need some adaptation to be able to be a more active participant in class games? Or is the child who has trouble speaking unable to demonstrate knowledge and express choices? Therefore, the specific tasks a child needs to complete will affect the choice of assistive technology solutions.

Consideration of relevant environmental issues: Technology solutions may also vary depending on the environments in which a child will use them. The environment of free play in a preschool or child care center may present different demands than a structured instructional setting. If the task being addressed by the technology relates to communication, the child may need to use the technology in many environments, including on the playground and at home.

Consideration of low-tech to high-tech options: Decisions about selecting appropriate assistive technology for young children should always consider the low-tech-to-high-tech continuum. Low-tech solutions should be considered first, before moving on to more expensive and complicated high-tech tools (Mistrett et al., 2006). This is in keeping with a basic principle in design and engineering—KISS: Keep It Short and Simple.

Provision of necessary supports: Parents and professionals will not be successful in their efforts to integrate assistive technology without adequate training and ongoing technical support (Dell, Newton, & Petroff, 2008; QIAT Consortium, 2005). They need hands-on training so that they become comfortable using the technology and teaching the child to use it effectively. Because technical problems are not unusual, assistive technology users also need to be able to access technical support in a timely fashion.

Use of assessment information: An assistive technology assessment is not an end point; rather, it should be viewed as the beginning of a cyclical process. Once assistive technology tools have been selected for a child, a trial period should ensue (Bowser & Reed, 1995). This is a time period in which professionals, parents, and the child experiment with the recommended technology. This is especially helpful in determining the feasibility of using the assistive technology in the child's natural environments. Following this trial period, the adequacy of the technology must be continually monitored. It is important to periodically reexamine the child's characteristics, tasks to be accomplished, and environments in which the child functions, because these often change over time. The assistive technology solutions that initially meet a child's needs may become inadequate or inappropriate as the child gets older and masters news skills and/or as the demands of the environments change.

SETT framework for decision making: A decision-making framework that is based on the above principles is Zabala's SETT Framework (2009). SETT is an acronym for Student, Environments, Tasks, and Tools. The team begins its discussion by delineating the student's (i.e., child's) needs and abilities. The team then brainstorms the various environments in which the child functions and the activities that take place in those environments. Only after these three issues are explored does the team consider specific assistive technology tools. In this way the focus remains on the child and the child's curricular goals.

TECHNOLOGY TOOLS TO SUPPORT EARLY INTERVENTION GOALS COMMUNICATION

Early communication development requires that children participate actively in their environment—through play, interactions with other children, and interactions with adults during daily routines, for example—and that they be provided with multiple opportunities to engage in communicative-rich environments with a variety of competent partners (Dell et al., 2008). However, social, cognitive, motor, and/or sensory disabilities often limit the accessibility of objects, people, communicative-rich environments, and opportunities. Many children with severe disabilities remain dependent on nonsymbolic behaviors as their primary system of communication (Ogletree, 1996). For example, they use facial grimaces to express dislikes, protest through the use of crying, or exhibit problematic behavior to communicate frustration.

Whereas typically developing children learn communication skills through typical daily interactions, children with significant disabilities often require direct, systematic instruction (Noonan & Siegel-Causey, 1997). They must be taught the fundamental concept that their actions can influence the environment and that deliberate interactions can achieve desired ends (i.e., cause and effect). Assistive technology can be harnessed to teach this fundamental concept to children with cognitive, motor, and sensory impairments. It offers solutions to the problem of providing these children with opportunities to communicate and make choices. Through the use of low-tech devices to request attention, develop understanding of consequences, and stimulate the sensory system, children with disabilities can be provided with opportunities to access environments rich in interesting objects and people (Dell et al., 2008).

Cause and Effect

Direct instruction in cause and effect can be provided through the use of simple switch technology. Switches enable children who have limited motor control to activate battery-operated toys and other electronic equipment with a single movement, such as flexing a fist or turning the head. They enable young children with disabilities to interact positively with their immediate surroundings and exert control over relevant stimuli (Lancioni et al., 2002; Langley, 1990). To adapt battery-operated toys, a small wafer-sized device called a battery adaptor is inserted in the toy's battery compartment between the battery leads. An adapted switch is plugged into the input jack at the other end. When the switch is depressed, the electrical circuit is complete, and the toy is activated. Any battery-operated toy or game can be adapted in this fashion (Levin & Scherfenberg, 1990).

Many different kinds of switches are available. Some switches are large and can be pressed with a fist, foot, or elbow. Others are tiny and require only a light touch; they can be activated with a single finger movement, a chin, or even a muscle twitch. Switches may be positioned and/or mounted in a variety of ways to facilitate activation. Wireless switches are also available.

It is therefore essential to involve a physical and/or occupational therapist when determining which switch will work most effectively with a child, the specific motor behavior that the child will use to activate it, and where and how the switch and the child should be positioned (York, Nietupski, & Hamre-Nietupski, 1985).

To teach cause and effect, a simple switch can be used to turn on a model race car that zooms around, makes car sounds, and flashes lights. For a child who is deaf/blind, a switch can activate a vibrating pillow that tickles. Switches can turn on a CD player that plays a child's favorite song or story. Each time the child presses the switch, the enjoyable consequence results.

Choice Making

This setup can be expanded easily to offer choice making. Choice making provides children with a sense of power and is an important developmental skill that must be exercised often, especially for the child who is still developing intentional communication (Dell et al., 2008). During free play, for example, a child can be provided with two switch setups—the race car mentioned above and a battery-operated pig that snorts and dances. Or the choice could be between listening to a favorite song or a favorite story on CD. All the child needs to do is hit the switch connected to the preferred object with a fist or other body part over which the child has control. To be effective, it is essential that these switch setups use toys, songs, and/or stories that are enjoyed by the individual child, not simply objects that are at hand. It is also essential that the choices be rotated so that the child is truly making a choice and not randomly hitting the switch.

Augmentative Communication

Moving on from promoting the prelinguistic skills of cause and effect and choice making to early communication, assistive technology offers a range of options. From simple single-message communicators to complex computerized devices, this technology is called augmentative and alternative communication (shortened here to augmentative communication). Augmentative communication is "any device, system, or method that improves the ability of a child with communication impairment to communicate effectively" (Pennsylvania Training and Technical Assistance Network, 2005, p. 5). Single-message communicators such as AbleNet's BIGmack or LITTLEmack look like switches but contain sound chips that can be recorded with spoken messages. Children can activate these prerecorded devices to initiate communication and/or respond to another person. For example, a child can invite another child to play a game by pressing a single message communicator that asks, "Would you like to play a game with me?" Or a child could ask an adult to read a book by pressing a LITTLEmack that says "Will you please read this book to me?" A child could participate in story time by using a single-message communicator to recite the refrain from a story (e.g., "But the caterpillar was still hungry"; Carle, 2007). Single-message communicators are often used as calling or alerting devices to enable children to request attention in an appropriate manner. Because messages can be recorded so quickly and easily, single-message communicators can be used to convey news from home, at circle time, or, if sent home with a child, news from school at home.

For slightly longer messages, devices called step-by-step communicators enable teachers and parents to record a series of messages. The child presses it once to speak the first message, again to speak the next message in the sequence, and so on. Step-by-step communicators are good choices for recording verses of a song or a poem, steps in a recipe, or short social scripts to encourage conversational turn-taking. The following profile of a 5-year old illustrates this application (Dell et al., 2008):

Peter is an outgoing and attentive 5-year old who attends a neighborhood preschool. He has cerebral palsy due to prematurity and his speech is unintelligible to most people. He uses a power wheelchair for mobility, which he controls with a set of switches. Peter's peers in his preschool attempt to interact with him, and he responds with smiles and vocalizations, but he rarely initiates an interaction. Since he does not have symbolic communication strategies, these interactions are usually brief and not sustained. A combination of several simple communication devices have been incorporated into Peter's preschool to foster his social interactions and provide opportunities for him to initiate communication.

- Peter uses a fist to activate a single-step communicator, which has been prerecorded by his brother, to greet his peers and ask questions. In the morning when he presses the device, it says, "Hey! Ask me what I did last night!" and he holds an object or picture that provides a hint, such as an advertisement for a DVD he had watched. Thus, a simple conversation can take place between Peter and his classmates.
- When Peter needs assistance, he calls the classroom aide with another single-step communicator that is programmed with the aide's name.
- During circle time, Peter uses a talking photo album from Radio Shack to share a weekend experience. He chooses among a sequence of three pictures, each of which has a message recorded

on its sound chip. When he activates each message it retells his experience. "We went fishing on Sunday!" "I hooked a really big fish!" "But it got away."

Single-message communicators and step-by-step communicators are valuable for early communicators and for teaching the power of communication. For children who need to express more than a few words, assistive technology offers a range of devices that are tailored to the needs of young children. They are lightweight for easy carrying and durable enough to withstand daily use. Many come with multiple layouts—for example, 4-, 8-, 16-, and 32-location display options—so the device's communication capacity can grow along with the child's skills. Others come with multiple levels so that the device can store more messages. The lower-priced devices, such as the Go-Talk (Attainment), use paper overlays that need to be changed as the child moves to a different level. Higher-priced devices such as the M3 (Dynavox) or the Springboard Lite (Prentke Romich) use dynamic display technology (i.e., touch screens) to change the visual display electronically. This technology offers the ability to store many messages in the device, providing a much larger vocabulary; the trick then becomes how to arrange them so children can find what they need quickly.

Augmentative Communication Decision Making

In addition to the characteristics of exemplary assistive technology assessments discussed in the section above, decisions about augmentative communication solutions need to consider three major components that make up any augmentative communication system: The *symbol system*, which is used to represent vocabulary, the specific *vocabulary* or messages the child will express with the system, and the method by which the child will *access* the system.

Symbol System

In selecting a symbol system, the team must determine which kind of symbols will be most understandable to the child. A symbol system can range from concrete systems such as real objects to abstract symbols, such as letters and words. In between are symbol systems comprised of photographs, line drawings, and icons. Symbol systems are classified according to their degree of "iconicity," that is, the clarity of their meanings in isolation (Beukelman & Mirenda, 2005). Photographs and real objects are said to be "transparent" because their meaning is clear without any additional information. Written words are considered "opaque" because they can be understood only by people who can read. In between, symbol sets are said to be "translucent" because the meanings of some of the symbols are obvious, but other symbols are more abstract; translucent symbol sets are usually comprised of line drawings. Beginning augmentative communicators usually need transparent symbols. Children learn to identify translucent symbols such as line drawings with some direct teaching.

Boardmaker (Mayer-Johnson) is a widely used software program that enables professionals and parents to create communication layouts using a symbol system that is based on line drawings (Picture Communication Symbols). Many of the symbols for common nouns and verbs are easily understood and are considered transparent; for example, Boardmaker's rendering of a dish of ice cream. Other symbols require some shared knowledge to understand; these are not as obvious and are considered translucent. The symbol for "football game," for example, is a picture of a football with two arrows facing each other. It is clear to the viewer that the symbol has something to do with football, but one needs some knowledge or training to recognize the symbol specifically as a football game. With a computer, a color printer, and the Boardmaker software, professionals and parents can easily create customized communication boards that can be used in a variety of settings.

For young children who need concrete symbols, technology offers two convenient options: (1) images downloaded from the Internet, and (2) digital photographs. By searching Google Images (http://images.google.com/) for a specific item, users can find good-quality photos of objects familiar to young children. For example, an exact image of a child's favorite toy or cookie can be found by searching Google Images. Digital cameras can be used to create concrete symbols of people in a child's life, rooms in a child's house, areas in a preschool, the family car, pets, and so forth.

Selecting Vocabulary

Once an appropriate symbol system and the device(s) are identified, an initial vocabulary must be selected. What messages would the child need and want to express to others? Selecting appropriate vocabulary is a critical factor in the successful use of any augmentative communication system (Balandin & Iacono, 1998; Beukelman & Mirenda, 2005). Teams often make the mistake of identifying vocabulary that is important to caregivers or teachers rather than messages that are relevant to the child who will be using the system. The team must make a concerted effort to identify vocabulary that is empowering to the child. This means selecting messages that are highly motivating, such as requests for preferred objects or activities, questions that will enable the child to initiate conversation with another child, and comments that will get a reaction from other people. The selection of specific words and phrases should fit with the child's culture and age group. Early intervention professionals need to become familiar with the slang in use in their location and incorporate these phrases in the device's vocabulary. Humor is often very motivating for children, so including jokes is often effective. Other guidelines for identifying meaningful vocabulary include the following:

- Provide messages that enable the child to greet other children and begin a conversation.
- Include vocabulary that enables the child to comment on events and activities, both as a way to express his or her opinion and as a way to continue a conversation. For example, "Pooh is so funny," "The wolf is scary," "That's gross!"
- Provide vocabulary that includes specific people who are important in the child's life and enables the child to call them.
- Make sure the child has a way of conveying his or her feelings, such as "That makes me really angry."
- Include a method for protest so the child has a way to refuse or say "NO." For example, "I don't want to do that."
- Use age-appropriate and culturally sensitive words and phrases, including slang.

Arranging Symbols

In addition to selecting the symbol system and the vocabulary, the collaborative team must decide how to arrange the symbols on the device. Since efficiency in communicating is the greatest challenge to an augmentative communication user, the arrangement of symbols should maximize the child's rate of communication. Preferred layouts include those that allow the child easy access to vocabulary that is likely to be used often and ease in constructing novel messages. A child who has control over only one hand, for example, needs frequently used words and phrases placed on the side of the device closest to his functioning hand. Decisions about symbol arrangement should take into consideration the child's developmental stage. For children whose language is still developing, a symbol array that provides practice in typical language skills may be helpful. For example, a child who is learning the rules of word order in sentences may benefit from a symbol array that groups parts of speech together—nouns on the left, verbs in the middle, adjectives on the right. As the child constructs a sentence, he or she moves from left to right, an essential skill in literacy development. Children who are learning about classifying items by attributes may need an array that groups categories of items together, such as food, toys, and family members (Beukelmen & Mirenda, 2005).

Visual Scene Display is a symbol arrangement that is effective with beginning communicators and those with complex challenges. Instead of simply arranging symbols in rows and columns, a visual scene display begins with a large picture or photograph that provides a context for more detailed information (Blackstone, 2004). As the child clicks on a part of the large picture, vocabulary related to that selection appears. For example, a picture of a kitchen is shown on the screen. When the child touches the image of a refrigerator, symbols related to juice, milk, fruit, and other favorite items found in the refrigerator are made visible. When the child touches the image of the kitchen table, vocabulary that could be used during family mealtimes is made visible. Using visual scene displays in augmentative communication devices creates a shared context for vocabulary. Research suggests it reduces the learning demands on young users and shifts the focus away from simple requests for desired objects to social interaction (Blackstone, 2004).

Access to the System

In addition to the symbol system and vocabulary selection, the team must consider how the child will access the vocabulary on the device. What parameters and challenges does the child present regarding access to the use of an augmentative communication device? Which access method will be most effective at this time? Physical therapists and occupational therapists are needed to contribute their knowledge about the child's motor abilities. Children who have a reliable point can use direct selection to construct messages on either low-tech language boards or high-tech computer-based systems. The point does not need to be with an index finger; if a child has more control over a thumb or fourth finger, for example, he or she can point with that digit (see Williams, 2006). The augmentative communication device will speak whatever symbols to which the child points.

For children who are unable to point with a finger, the team will need to consider other access methods. Direct selection may also be accomplished with a joystick, a low-tech pointing device such as a dowel held in a child's fist, or a head stick attached with a headband. A joystick is a good choice when a child has enough motor control to maneuver it in at least four directions and hit a button or switch to make a selection. A candidate for a dowel held in a fist is a child who has control of large arm movements without control of a single digit. A possible candidate for a head stick is a child whose head control is better than his or her hand/arm control. A high-tech access method for a child who has decent head control involves an infrared beam that is mounted on a child's eyeglasses, hat, or headband. Both low-tech and high-tech head pointing systems work best when the child has good vision and is able to move his or her head in small increments for precise positioning. High-tech head pointing systems also require the user to be able to keep his or her head still when necessary.

Eye gaze systems are a high-tech access method that utilizes the movements of a child's eyes. Eye gaze systems use infrared-sensitive video cameras to determine the precise spot on a display at which a child is looking. Selecting a symbol is accomplished by activating a switch, blinking the eye, or simply dwelling on the desired item. The augmentative communication system will speak whatever symbols the child selects. Because eye gaze systems require extensive training and positioning and are expensive, they are appropriate for young children only when communication is not accessible to the child with any other access method.

For children who do not have adequate head control or finger/hand control, augmentative communication is still accessible via an access method called single-switch scanning. Using a switch such as those discussed above, single-switch scanning requires reliable control over only a single movement such as flexing a fist, turning a head to one side, or moving a knee. The child watches the screen as an electric highlighter moves from symbol to symbol. When the highlighter reaches the symbol that the child desires, the child activates the switch to select the item and the augmentative communication device speaks the selection. Although single-switch scanning is extremely slow, it is an important access method because it is often the *only* means by which a child with severe physical disabilities can access communication.

Variations of these access methods can also be used to control a power wheelchair. If a child already has a reliable method for accessing his or her wheelchair, a similar method should be considered for the augmentative communication system. This is an example of the importance of the team approach to assistive technology decision making.

Myths about Augmentative Communication

Although the research clearly documents the benefits of augmentative communication, and many first-person accounts attest to its indispensable role in the lives of the writers, its adoption in early intervention has been hampered by a lingering of outdated myths among professionals and parents (Romski & Sevcik, 2005). It is important to examine these misconceptions and counter them with accurate information so that professionals and parents will be open to the possibility of introducing augmentative communication supports to young children who could benefit from them.

Myth #1: Augmentative communication will inhibit further development of speech. Too many professionals and parents are under the false impression that if a child is provided with an augmentative communication system, the child will lose the motivation to speak and will cease trying. The empirical research shows the exact opposite (Romski & Sevcik, 2005; Schlosser, 2003). Augmentative communication interventions have been shown to enhance the development of speech in children who have adequate oral-motor control (Cress, 2003). This makes logical sense because speech is the most efficient form of expressive language; augmentative communication is slow, and even the most skilled augmented communicator cannot reach the speeds of typical speakers.

Myth #2: Augmentative communication should be used only as a last resort. This myth is closely linked to Myth #1 and stems from a set of beliefs from the early days of augmentative communication that have since been discredited (Schlosser, 2003). The use of augmentative and alternative communication interventions (AAC) "should not be contingent on failure to develop speech skills or considered a last resort because AAC can play many roles in early communication development. . . . In fact, it is critical that AAC be introduced before communication failure occurs" (Romski & Sevcik, 2005, pp. 178–179).

Myth #3: A child must demonstrate a set of prerequisite skills before augmentative communication can be introduced. There are no readiness criteria for teaching communication (Beukelman & Mirenda, 2005). Waiting for children to be "ready" only serves to prevent the development of needed communication skills. Young children with severe sensory, physical, or multiple disabilities may not be able to demonstrate cognitive abilities without a means of communication (Romski & Sevcik, 2005). To deny them augmentative communication because they do not display a cognitive skill that they cannot demonstrate without augmentative communication is senseless and potentially damaging circular reasoning.

Myth #4: Augmentative communication requires some level of literacy prior to consideration. Literacy skills are not needed to use and/or learn to use augmentative communication systems. In fact, the research demonstrates that augmentative communication devices can actually provide a *means* to further develop literacy skills (Erickson, 2000; Hetzroni, 2004; Musselwhite & King-DeBaun, 1997).

Assistive Technology to Support Play

Providing access to and increasing participation in developmentally appropriate play is another benefit of using assistive technology in early intervention settings (Hamm, Mistrett, & Goetz Ruffino, 2006). Assistive technology can facilitate toy exploration (Burkhart, n.d.), art activities (Dinse, n.d.), participation in group games, and music making. It can provide alternative means for children with disabilities to interact with their environment, toys, other children, and adults.

For example, low-tech solutions can make puzzle play accessible to young children who have delays in fine motor skills. Pieces of dowels can be glued to puzzle pieces so children who do not have a pincer grasp can manipulate puzzle pieces with a palmer grasp. Place mats made out of nonslip material like Dycem will help keep toys and all their component pieces in place for children who lack fine motor control. Velcro glued to blocks is another low-tech solution for children with motor control problems.

Art activities such as drawing, coloring, and painting can also be supported with low-tech solutions. A clipboard can be used to stabilize the paper for a child who cannot use both hands. Some children may have better control using a slant board to hold their paper at a 15- to 30-degree angle; adults can easily devise a slant board by gluing a clipboard to a large plastic three-ring binder. Children who have a whole-hand grasp can use rubber stamps to create pictures. Utensil grips made out of clay or foam (or purchased) can be used to build up the handles of crayons, markers, paintbrushes, and rubber stamps. Painting mittens are useful for children who cannot grasp at all and for children who are tactilely defensive (Dinse, n.d.).

Assistive technology using adapted switches enable young children with physical, cognitive, and multiple disabilities to partially participate in play activities. Although the severity of their disabilities may prevent them from performing in every part of the activity, technology can involve them to some extent. For example, a child who cannot ambulate for a game of musical chairs can still participate in the game by using a switch to turn the music (CD, tape, or MP3 player) on and off. A child who cannot squeeze the paint bottles to create a spin-art picture can use a switch to turn on the spinner for the other children (Levin & Scherfenberg, 1990). There are even battery-operated water guns that can be controlled with a switch.

Switches can be used to activate battery-operated race cars, trains, singing and dancing animals, talking robots, and talking Christmas trees, to name a few. The key to selecting from the wide range of available battery-operated toys is that the child must *like* the toy he or she will be playing with. Children will be motivated to activate the switch when the result is enjoyable.

Electronic "busy boxes" or activity centers that have already been adapted are available from assistive technology vendors such as Enabling Devices (http://enablingdevices.com). Designed to provide sensory stimulation to children with multiple disabilities, these activity centers offer tactile feedback such as textured pads, vibrating plates, and fans that blow air, as well as blinking lights, visual effects, and sound effects.

With developmentally appropriate software programs, computers offer high-tech options for engaging young children in play activities. (Many software programs are now Web-based, meaning they are played directly on the Internet instead of from a CD or hard drive. The term "software" will be used to refer to activities played on a computer, whether they are housed on a CD, hard drive, or the Internet.) Computer technology is especially powerful as a tool for play because it is flexible, adaptable, responsive, and engaging. Many companies offer interactive activities on their Web sites that use characters from favorite children's movies and television shows. Although adults may not warm to these, children are drawn to them and are quickly engaged in activities that include them.

The commercial software market changes so rapidly that there is no point in recommending specific software titles in this chapter. However, a discussion of desirable features of software for young children will provide guidance on how to select computer-based activities for young children. Since most young children are nonreaders, they need software that that speaks all instructions and reads text aloud.

Children with attention problems or visual impairments need a consistent, uncluttered visual display so they are not distracted or confused by sensory overload (Dell & Newton, 1998). The activities need to be untimed—i.e., self-paced—so children have time to think, make choices, and move without the pressure of a ticking clock. This is especially important for children who have delays in motor development. Feedback needs to be consistent, unambiguous, and appropriate to the task; it should be helpful or neutral, not distracting. Most importantly, the software needs to provide options for teachers and parents to customize it for individual children. For example, for children who are overstimulated by auditory stimuli, it is important to be able to turn the sound off. If the program is designed to encourage young children to explore letters and letter sounds, it is helpful if it offers an option to choose upper- or lowercase letters (Dell & Newton, 1998).

One of the most valuable aspects of using computer technology with young children is that it can make play activities accessible to children whose disabilities preclude them from participating in typical play activities. A child who cannot physically explore, sort, or manipulate objects may be able to participate in comparable activities on a computer. A child who cannot manipulate a crayon or marker can create pictures using a graphics program like KidPix Studio Deluxe (Riverdeep). To do this, teachers and parents need to determine if the child can interact with a computer using a standard keyboard and mouse or if the child needs an alternative method to access the computer.

Young children with decent motor control often respond well to touch screens. They can make selections and move items just by touching, with no intermediate step. Another option is an adapted trackball; this works like a mouse but is much easier to manipulate and provides simple buttons in place of double-click and click-and-drag functions. Expanded keyboards—large keyboards with large keys, sometimes arranged in an alphabetical array—may be appropriate for children who can point but lack fine motor control and/or are confused by a standard QWERTY keyboard. Customizable keyboards such as Intelli-Keys enable teachers and parents to design the content and appearance of each key. For example, an adult could design an overlay with pictures and greetings appropriate for a birthday card, and the child could create birthday cards for his family by simply pressing the keys of his choice. This is especially helpful for a child who can only use a fist or a child who has severe attention problems. Additional information on accessing computerized devices is provided above in the section on communication.

Play activities for young children that can be facilitated by assistive technology also include cause-and-effect-type toys, communication, and early literacy activities. These applications of assistive technology are discussed separately in this chapter.

Assistive Technology to Support Daily Routines

Whether a child is using a single-message communicator, a cardboard communication board, or a high-tech device, augmentative communication technology can be used to enable the child to communicate choices and opinions during daily routines in natural environments. Professionals and parents must seek every opportunity for young children to practice their communication skills and conduct conversations throughout the day. They need to provide deliberate interventions that support the use of augmentative communication systems and the development of communication. Using the context of daily routines and naturally occurring events, in both home and intervention environments, is recognized as a powerful approach to communication skill development. A specific protocol for this practice, Environmental Communication Teaching (ECT; Karlan, 1991; Mervine, 1995), focuses on identifying the communication demands of natural environments, teaching parents and professionals to prompt communication efforts, and systematically arranging to expand communication exchanges.

Young children's daily routines provide a perfect opportunity to encourage communication. Morning routines, for example, provide regular opportunities for a child to choose which item of clothing to wear. "I want to wear the green one" and "I want to wear the red one" could be programmed into any of the devices discussed above. Or a "dressing" communication board could be designed in *Boardmaker*, slid into a clear sheet protector, and hung in a child's bedroom. The child could point to the color and/or type of item he or she wishes to wear each day. In cold climates, for example, the child could choose between wearing a sweatshirt and wearing a sweater. During bedtime routines, a child could choose which pajamas to wear or which stuffed toy to take to bed.

Mealtimes present similar opportunities for communication (PACER Center, 2006). Messages such as "please," "thank you," "May I have more," and "I'm full" can be included in the augmentative communication device's vocabulary as can a family's grace before meals. The child's favorite foods should be added to the device so they can be requested. Mealtimes are also the occasion for social interactions and, as such, provide a good opportunity to practice relevant vocabulary.

"I played with the blocks today," "I painted a picture," "I heard a funny story," and "I played in the sandbox" are examples of messages that could be selected to answer a parent's question, "What did you do today?"

In school, daily routines such as arrival and dismissal, circle time, and snack (or lunch) time, present similar opportunities for communication. Single-message communicators can be hung in various places around the room so several children can access them—"Good morning" near the classroom door in the morning, "Bye! See you tomorrow" in the afternoon, "Want to play?" in the block area, and "Would you read this book to me?" in the library corner. A single-message communicator can also be used to enable a child to participate in singing the morning song. Vocabulary on multi-message devices should provide opportunities for the child to utilize a variety of communicative functions in addition to greeting other people, making requests, and answering questions, such as commenting on activities and events ("That's funny!" "That's scary"), expressing emotions ("I'm mad!" "I love you"), and rejecting or protesting ("I don't want to do that," "Leave me alone").

Other kinds of assistive technology can be used to facilitate young children's participation in daily routines. Small grooming appliances like an electric toothbrush and a hair dryer can be adapted so that children can turn them on with a switch (Mistrett et al., 2006; Levin & Scherfenberg, 1990). Battery-operated appliances are adapted and connected to a switch in the same way as battery-operated toys. Using switches to turn on electrical devices that run on 120 volts requires an additional piece of equipment called a PowerLink control unit (AbleNet). The appliance's power cord plugs into an outlet on the PowerLink, and a switch is inserted into its input jack. The appliance's on/off switch is left in the "on" position, but the appliance will not be turned on until the child hits the switch. These setups enable young children with physical and/or cognitive disabilities to partially participate in daily activities. Children can use a switch to turn on an electric mixer during a baking activity at home, or a popcorn popper to make snacks for the family or classmates (Levin & Scherfenberg, 1990).

Early and Emergent Literacy

The behaviors of reading and writing begin to develop at a very young age, much earlier than was previously realized, and the research shows that written and oral language develop concurrently (Sulzby

& Teale, 1991). This means that the practice of waiting for children to develop expressive communication before introducing literacy activities is a mistake and puts children with disabilities at an even greater disadvantage (Koppenhaver & Yoder, 1993).

For children with severe disabilities, the motor, cognitive, and sensory impairments that interfere with their communication development also interfere with their access to early reading and writing activities (Dell et al., 2008). Children who cannot speak are frequently not viewed as literate, and as a result, are not provided with opportunities to experience early reading and writing activities. Therefore, it is essential that young children with severe disabilities be actively engaged in activities that promote emergent literacy (Erickson & Koppenhaver, 1995; Light & McNaughton, 1993; Musselwhite & King-DeBaun, 1997). These children need environments that are rich in both spoken language and the printed word, and they need multiple opportunities to handle books (e.g., orient the book, turn the pages) and interact with print (Hutinger, Bell, Daytner, & Johanson, 2006). In this way, they learn the conventions of print, such as reading from left to right and from front cover to back cover. Early literacy activities enable young children to see the connection between the words on the page and the stories that are read to them (Lewis & Tolla, 2003). Many children with severe disabilities need direct and deliberate instruction in early literacy skills (Musslewhite & King-DeBaun, 1997).

Both switch and augmentative communication technology can be harnessed to provide opportunities for young children with disabilities to engage in literacy-focused activities. Low-tech solutions include making simple slant boards and book stabilizers using carpet, three-ring binders, and Velcro (Spring, 2004). A variety of materials can be attached to book pages with a hot-melt glue gun to create "page fluffers" that keep the pages separate and enable a child with limited motor control to turn the page (Musslewhite & King-DeBaun, 1997). For children who are blind or visually impaired, real objects representing the story can be glued to the pages as tactile cues or collected in a ziplock bag and attached to the book (Lewis & Tolla, 2003). A piece of blanket-like fabric, for example, can be glued to the page in which Goldilocks tries out the bears' beds and a piece of dry cereal where she tastes the oatmeal. Single-message communicators can be set up to recite the refrain of a story so a child can participate in the choral part of story-telling (e.g., "He huffed and he puffed and he blew the house in!"). Step-by-step communicators can be recorded with sequential refrains.

Board books that talk are now widely available commercially. When a child presses a designated button, a sentence corresponding to the picture on the page is read aloud. An assistive technology device called a BookWorm (AbleNet) can convert any book into a talking book. The BookWorm uses sound chip technology to provide up to eight minutes of recorded speech and provides a button on a strip to correspond to each page. An adult simply attaches a removable sticker to each page of a child's favorite book and records the story, page by page. The child can then listen to the story by pressing on the button that corresponds to each sticker. These low-tech adaptations enable children with disabilities to begin to handle books, interact with print, and listen to the rhythms of spoken stories.

Young children can listen to stories and children's books on CD or on MP3 players (e.g., the Apple iPod) while they follow along in the actual book. A CD player can be adapted so that a child can start and stop it with a single switch. Many children's books' titles are available for download as digital audio files on Internet sites like Project Gutenberg (http://www.gutenberg.net) and Bookshare (http://www.bookshare .org). These files can be transferred to a portable MP3 player so children can listen to them without being tethered to a computer. Video streaming is another technology that offers read-aloud stories. For example, Story-line Online (http://www.storylineonline.net), a Web site run by the Screen Actors Guild Foundation, presents videos of actors and actresses reading favorite children's books aloud while showing the words and illustrations.

Software programs offer high-tech solutions to engaging young children in early literacy activities. Hutinger et al. (2006) categorized early literacy software into three types: (1) interactive literacy-based software, such as the Living Books (Riverdeep) series; (2) graphics and story-making software, such as Kid Pix Studio Deluxe (Riverdeep) and Storybook Weaver Deluxe (Riverdeep); and (3) authoring programs, such as IntelliTools's Classroom Suite, which can be used by teachers and parents to create their own stories based on children's individual experiences. Interactive literacy-based software programs convert popular children's books from the standard presentation of text with pictures in a bound book to a multimedia display that reads the text aloud, provides music and sound effects, and offers young readers opportunities to make things happen on the screen. These software programs also allow children to control the timing and repetition of words and sentences (Hutinger et al. 2006). Using a mouse or trackball, children need only click on pictures or words on the screen to cause the program to react. If used with a touch screen, these programs will react with a simple pointing on the screen. Adaptations are available that will make these programs accessible to children who use single switches.

Graphics and story-making software are software programs that enable children to create pictures and stories of their own design. Using whatever access method they need, children can choose pictures, colors, letters, sounds, clips of music, etc., arrange them on the screen, and manipulate them. This type of program empowers young children to create pictures and storybooks that far exceed their abilities to draw and write. For children who cannot hold a crayon or paintbrush due to physical disabilities, this type of program enables them to produce a creative work that would be impossible without technology.

Simple authoring programs like My Own Bookshelf (SoftTouch) enable teachers and parents to create interactive stories that children can access on computers. The computer reads aloud the text while displaying whatever pictures the teacher or parent has selected for the book. In addition to offering the opportunity to create stories that relate to a child's specific experiences, this technology enables parents and teachers to write stories that *include* the child in it (by importing photos from a digital camera).

Teachers and parents can also create simple switch-accessible talking books using Microsoft PowerPoint, a software program with which many people are already familiar (Spring, 2004). Step-by-step instructions are available on the following Web sites: http://www.cast.org (Center for Applied Special Technology), http://www.setbc.org (Special Education Technology–British Columbia), and http://atto.buffalo.edu (Assistive Technology Training Online Project at the University of Buffalo). Anybody with basic computer skills should be able to create a talking book following these instructions. It is recommended that professionals and parents spend a little time creating a template so that they can produce several books more quickly (i.e., by just changing the text and pictures).

FUTURE TRENDS

As technology becomes further entrenched in our society, its price tag continues to decline, and empirical evidence demonstrates its effectiveness, assistive technology is likely to be used more and more in early intervention. However, the challenge will be to seamlessly integrate it into the early intervention curriculum and not treat it simply as an add-on (FCTD, 2007). Adequate training and technical support for teachers and parents will be critical. Preservice preparation of early intervention personnel will need to incorporate appropriate applications of assistive technology so the field will be staffed by knowledgeable practitioners. There is a particular need for speech-language pathologists who are aware of and skilled in leading the selection and design of augmentative communication systems for young children.

Commercially available toys and technology in the near future are likely to adhere to the principles of universal design (FCTD, 2007). Universal design is "the design of products and environments to be usable by all people, to the greatest extent possible, without the need for adaptation or specialized design" (Center for Universal Design, 1997, para. 3). Before a product or environment is developed and marketed, universal design recommends considering "the needs of the greatest number of possible users, [thereby] eliminating the need for costly, inconvenient, and unattractive adaptations later on" (CAST, 2006). This concept began in the field of architecture, then broadened to the fields of hardware and software development, and is now a key principle in instructional design.

Two popular conveniences today illustrate the concept of universal design: automatic doors and curb cuts. Automatic doors make stores, airports, and other public spaces accessible to individuals with disabilities, but they also make those places accessible to a broader range of people: shoppers pushing shopping carts, travelers wheeling suitcases, parents pushing children in strollers, elderly people, and others who lack the strength to open heavy doors. Curb cuts were originally designed to make navigating city streets more accessible to wheelchair users, but they turned out to benefit many more people—workers making deliveries with hand trucks, elderly people using walkers, roller bladers, and skateboarders, as well as people pulling city shopping baskets and pushing baby strollers. In sum, automatic doors and curb cuts benefit a wide range of people, including individuals with disabilities.

Toy manufacturers and software publishers have begun applying this principle to the development of toys and software. Many products are now available that are flexible and easily adaptable to be used by the widest range of children. This trend is evident in the *Let's Play Toy Guide* (2006) that was developed by the Toy Industry Foundation in partnership with the Alliance for Technology Access (ATA) and the American Foundation for the Blind (AFB). The toys listed in the guide are available commercially and were selected based on the toy's play value for children with disabilities. Many of the toys have large buttons and thick handles, which make them accessible to children with motor delays. Others talk or provide sound effects and/or blinking lights, features that may be engaging to children with sensory impairments and/or attention difficulties. This blurring of the line between specialized devices designed specifically for children with disabilities and commercially produced toys is likely to continue. The benefit to families is that commercial toys are less expensive and easier to find than toys produced by assistive technology companies.

A similar change is happening in computers, assistive technology devices, and augmentative communication devices. Touch screens, which in years past were specialized items available only through assistive technology vendors, are now mainstream technology. Tablet PCs, which are laptops that utilize touch-screen technology, are likely to become commonplace in early intervention programs. Children will be able to interact with computer games and activities by simply pointing to items on the screen. Teachers and speech-language therapists will be able to create talking communication boards without having to spend thousands of dollars on a dedicated augmentative communication device.

A related trend is that technology tools will continue to get smaller and more portable. Instead of having their children play on a tablet PC, some early intervention programs will utilize the touch-screen technology on an iPod Touch (or similar device). We will probably see an expansion of iPhones being used for augmentative communication. Increases in portability will also mean more wireless technology and longer-lasting batteries.

With the advent of Web 2.0 (i.e., the second generation of the World Wide Web) have come changes in how computer games and educational software are provided and how children interact with them. Buying children's games on CDs is fast becoming a thing of the past as computerized games and interactive educational activities increasingly reside on the Web (Bull & Ferster, 2005). Early intervention programs will purchase subscriptions to content. This means they will need to have fast and reliable Internet access. It also means that computers will continue to get smaller, since so much of the software being used will not need to be stored on the computer itself. An important benefit of Web 2.0 is that applications appropriate for young children will be available from *any* computer—any computer in the building, in another site, or in children's homes. Families will be able to play with their children on the same activities at home as in school. All of this means that timely and skilled training and technical support will be more essential than ever.

SUMMARY

When carefully selected and matched to an individual child's needs and environments, assistive technology has an important role to play in supporting the goals of early intervention. It can be harnessed to teach communication, cause and effect, and choice-making skills. With appropriate selection of vocabulary, it can be used as a means of augmentative communication for children who cannot speak. It can support play activities, facilitate participation in daily routines, and contribute to the development of early literacy. Since the world of computer technology changes so rapidly, it is impossible to predict how future applications will further benefit early intervention, but one thing is certain—new developments will bring with them exciting possibilities for young children with special needs.

References

Alliance for Technology Access. (2004). *Computer resources for people with disabilities* (4th ed.). Alameda, CA: Hunter House.

Alliance for Technology Access. (2006). *Let's play: A guide to toys for children with special needs.* Retrieved June 30, 2009, from http://www.afb.org/Section.asp?SectionID=62

Arnold, A. (2003). Augcomm user trouble-shoots for Prentke Romich Co. *TECH-NJ, 14*(1). Retrieved June 28, 2009, from http://www.tcnj.edu/~technj/2003/arnold

Balandin, S., & Iacono, T. (1998) A few well-chosen words. *Augmentative and Alternative Communication, 14,* 147–161.

Beukelman, D. R., & Mirenda, P. (2005). *Augmentative and alternative communication* (3rd ed.). Baltimore: Paul H. Brookes.

Blackstone, S. W. (2004, August). Visual scene displays. *ACN: Augmentative Communication News, 16*(2).

Bowser, G., & Reed, P. (1995). Education Tech Points for Assistive Technology Planning, *Journal of Special Education Technology, 12*(4), 325–338.

Bryant, B. R., Bryant, D. P., & Rieth, H. J. (2002). The use of assistive technology in postsecondary education. In L. Brinckerhoff, J. McGuire, & S. Shaw (Eds.) *Postsecondary education and transition for students with learning disabilities* (pp. 389–429). Austin, TX: Prod-Ed.

Bull, G., & Ferster, B. (2005). Ubiquitous computing in a Web 2.0 world. *Learning and Leading with Technology*, December–January, pp. 9–11. Retrieved July 7, 2009, from http://www.iste.org

Burkhart, L. (n.d.). What we are learning about early learners and augmentative communication and assistive technology. Retrieved July 29, 2009, from http://www.lburkhart.com

Carle, E. (2007). *The very hungry caterpillar*. New York: Philomel.

Center on Applied Special Technology (CAST). (2006). Research and development in universal design for learning. Retrieved June 30, 2009, from http://www.cast.org/research/index.html

Center for Universal Design. (1997). *About universal design*. Retrieved June 30, 2009, from http://www.design.ncsu.edu/cud/about_ud/about_ud.htm

Collins, R. (n.d.) *Independence can be cheap and easy with low tech assistive technology*. Retrieved June 28, 2009, from the Arizona Technology Access Program (AzTAP) Web site: http://www4.nau.edu/ihd/AzTAP/Initiative_on_Aging/AzTAP_AssistiveTechnologyandAginginPlace_Article2.asp

Cress, C. J. (2003). Responding to a common early childhood question: "Will my child talk?" *Perspectives on Augmentative and Alternative Communication, 12*, 10–11.

Dell, A. G., Newton, D. A., & Petroff, J. G. (2008). *Assistive technology in the classroom: Enhancing the school experiences of students with disabilities*. Upper Saddle River, NJ: Pearson/Merrill/Prentice Hall.

Dell, A. G., & Newton, D. A. (1998). Software for play and active early learning. *Exceptional Parent, 28*(11), 39–43.

Dinse, P. (n.d.). Assistive technology and peer socialization in early childhood special education. Retrieved June 28, 2009, from the AT Network Web site: http://www.atnet.org

Erickson, K. A. (2000). All children are ready to learn: An emergent versus readiness perspective in early literacy assessment. *Seminars in Speech and Language, 213*, 193–203.

Erickson, K. A., & Koppenhaver, D. A. (1995). Developing a literacy program for children with severe disabilities. *Reading Teacher, 48*, 8, 676–684.

Family Center on Technology and Disability (FCTD) (2007). Assistive technology and early childhood education: Capturing the teaching moment [interview with Linda Robinson], *FCTD News and Notes, 60*, 7. Retrieved July 24, 2009 from http://www.fctd.info/resources/newsletters/index.php

Fried-Oken, M., & Bersani, H. (Eds.). (2000). *Speaking up and spelling it out*. Baltimore: Paul H. Brookes.

Hamm, E. M., Mistrett, S. G., & Goetz Ruffino, A. (2006). Play outcomes and satisfaction with toys and technology of young children with special needs. *Journal of Special Education Technology, 21*(1).

Hetzroni, O. E. (2004). AAC and literacy. *Disability and Rehabilitation, 26*(21–22), 1305–1312.

Hutinger, P., Bell, C., Daytner, G., & Johanson, J. (2006). Establishing and maintaining an early childhood emergent literacy technology curriculum. *Journal of Special Education Technology, 21*(4), 39–54.

Individuals with Disabilities Education Act (IDEA) of 2004, 20 U.S.C. § 1401D.

Karlan, G. (1991). *Environmental communication teaching training*. Field-initiated research grant award No. H023C9005 from the Office of Special Education, U.S. Department of Education. Lafayette, IN: Purdue University.

Knezek, G., Christensen, R., Bell, L., & Bull, G. (2006). Identifying key research issues. *Learning and Leading with Technology, 33*(8), 18–20.

Koppenhaver, D., & Yoder, D. (1993). Classroom literacy instruction for children with severe speech and physical impairments (SSPI): What is and what might be? *Topics in Language Disorders, 13*, 1–15.

Langley, M. B. (1990). A developmental approach to the use of toys for facilitation of environmental control. *Physical and Occupational Therapy in Pediatrics, 10*, 69–91.

Lancioni, G. E., O'Reilly, M. F., Singh, N. N., Oliva, D., Piazzolla, G., Pirani, P., & Growneweg, J. (2002). Evaluating the use of multiple microswitches and responses for children with multiple disabilities. *Journal of Intellectual Disability Research, 46*(4), 346–351.

Levin, J., & Scherfenberg, L. (1990). *Selection and use of simple technology in home, school, work and community settings*. Minneapolis: AbleNet.

Lewis, S., & Tolla, J. (2003, January–February). Creating and using tactile experience books for young children with visual impairments. *Teaching Exceptional Children, 35*(3), 22–28.

Light, J., & McNaughton, D. (1993). Literacy and augmentative and alternative communication (AAC): The expectations and priorities of parents and teachers. *Topics in Language Disorders, 13*(2), 33–46.

Male, M. (2003). *Technology for inclusion: Meeting the needs of all students*. Boston: Allyn & Bacon.

Mervine, P. (1995). Teaching communication in natural environments. *TECH-NJ, 6* (1), 3, 16.

Mistrett, S., Ruffino, A., Lane, S., Robinson, L., Reed, P., & Milbourne, S. (2006). *Technology Supports for Young Children* [TAM Technology Fan]. Arlington, VA: Technology and Media Division (TAM).

Musselwhite, C., & King-DeBaun, P. (1997). *Emerging literacy success: Merging whole language and technology for students with disabilities*. Park City, UT: Creative Communicating.

National Organization on Disability. (2006). Economic participation: Technology. Retrieved July 28, 2009, from http://www.nod.org/index.cfm?fuseaction =page.viewPage&pageId=16

Nolet, V. & McLaughlin, M. J. (2000). *Accessing the general curriculum: Including students with disabilities in standards-based reform*. Thousand Oaks, CA: Corwin Press.

Noonan, M. J., & Siegel-Causey, E. (1997). Special needs of young children with severe handicaps. In L. McCormick, D. Loeb, & R. L. Schiefelbusch (Eds.). *Supporting children with communication difficulties in inclusive settings: School-based language intervention* (pp. 405–432). Boston: Allyn & Bacon.

Ogletree, B. T. (1996). Assessment targets and protocols for nonsymbolic communicators with profound disabilities. *Focus on Autism and Other Development Disabilities, 11*(1).

PACER Center. (2006). *EZ AT—Assistive technology activities for children ages 3–8 with disabilities: A guide for professionals and parents*. Minneapolis, MN: Author. Retrieved July 6, 2009, from http://www.pacer.org/publications/stc.asp

Pennsylvania Training and Technical Assistance Network (PaTTAN). (2005). *Assistive technology resource pack for early intervention families and professionals: Frequently asked questions*. Harrisburg, PA: Author. Retrieved June 22, 2009, from http://www.pattan.net/Publications.aspx?ContentLocation=/supportingstudents/AssistiveTechnology.aspx

QIAT Consortium. (2005). Quality Indicators for Assistive Technology services: Research-based revisions. Retrieved July 28, 2009, from http://www.qiat.org

Romski, M., & Sevcik, R. A. (2005). Augmentative communication and early intervention: Myths and realities. *Infants and Young Children, 18*(3), 174–185.

Salend, S. J. (2004). *Creating inclusive classrooms: Effective and reflective practices* (5th ed.) Columbus, OH: Merrill/Prentice Hall.

Schlosser, R. (2003). Effects of augmentative communication on natural speech development. In R. Schlosser, *The efficacy of augmentative and alternative communication: Toward evidence-based practice* (pp. 404–426). San Diego, CA: Academic Press.

Spring, D. (2004). Assistive technology supports for early childhood literacy. Retrieved July 22, 2009, from Michigan's Assistive Technology Resource (MATR): http://www.ecac-parentcenter.org/childhood/documents/AssistiveTech.pdf

Sulzby, E., & Teale, W. (1991). Emergent literacy. In R. Barr, M. L. Kamil, P. B. Mosenthal, & P. D. Pearson (Eds.), *Handbook of reading research* (vol. 2, pp. 727–757). New York: Longman.

Villa, R. A., & Thousand, J. S. (Eds.). (2000). *Restructuring for caring and effective education: Piecing the puzzle together* (2nd ed.). Baltimore: Paul H. Brookes.

Williams, M. (2006). *How far we've come, how far we've got to go: Tales from the AAC trenches*. DVD. Monterey, CA: Augmentative Communication, Inc.

York, J., Nietupski, J., & Hamre-Nietupski, S. (1985). A decision-making process for using microswitches. *Journal of the Association for Persons with Severe Handicaps, 10*(4), 214–223.

Zabala, J. (2009). SETT Framework. Retrieved January 25, 2010 from http://www.joyzabala.com

Chapter 6

Evidence-Based Practice in Early Childhood Intervention

Dale Walker

R esearch supporting early childhood intervention practice has grown extensively over the last 40 years (e.g., Guralnick, 1997; Huston, 2008; National Research Council & Institute of Medicine, 2000; Shonkoff & Meisels, 2000; Smith et al., 2002; Wolery & Bailey, 2002). Beginning research in early intervention and early childhood special education was primarily concerned with demonstrating the necessity for intervening early in life (National Research Council & Institute of Medicine, 2000). A number of early intervention programs designed to improve the developmental outcomes of at-risk children emphasized the importance of high-quality child care and preschool experiences to positive schooling outcomes—e.g., Abecedarian Project (Ramey & Campbell, 1992); CARE (Wasik, Ramey, Bryant, & Sparling, 1991); and Consortium for Longitudinal Studies (Lazar, Darlington, Murray, Royce, & Snipper, 1982). These programs provided intensive, comprehensive interventions to disadvantaged infants, young children, and their families with the purpose of demonstrating that early intervention could improve later developmental and school outcomes (Warren & Walker, 2005).

Once it was mandated under P.L. 99-457, the amendment of the Individual With Disabilities Education Act (IDEA) passed in 1986, that young children with disabilities were to receive educational services (U.S. Department of Education, Office of Special Education Programs, OSEP), the emphasis of early intervention research shifted to documenting how many children were actually being served. The field has since progressed beyond defending the importance of intervening early or marking success exclusively in terms of the numbers of children being served, to measuring the integrity of early intervention practice and effects on child outcomes.

WHY THE EMPHASIS ON EVIDENCE-BASED PRACTICE?

Leading to the emphasis on evidence-based practice in early childhood, early childhood special education has been legislative and policy mandates and recommendations including the Government Performance and Results Act (GPRA; Senate Committee on Governmental Affairs) calling for increased accountability for agencies receiving federal and state support (Office of Management and Budget [OMB], 2006). Foundations and other agencies have also required that agencies receiving funds be accountable for having an impact on children and families (Harbin, Rous, & McLean, 2005). Reporting of child and family outcomes, for example, is now required for all infants and young children with disabilities (Hebbeler, Barton, & Mallik, 2008), and educational policy emphasizes using scientifically based practices as mandated through the Individuals with Disabilities Education Act (IDEA, 2004) and No Child Left Behind (2001; Bruder, 2010; Buysse & Wesley, 2006; Huston, 2008). These, and other federal, state, and policy initiatives (e.g., Education Sciences Reform Act of 2002; Head Start Act of 1998) along with recommendations calling for accountability in early intervention and early childhood special education (EI/ECSE) have been established to ensure that young children with disabilities receive high-quality intervention and education that promotes their development and prepares them for success in their social relationships, in school, and in their community. There are however, few repositories of evidence-based practices from which early interventionists and educators can access the information needed to comply with mandates to use evidence-based practice.

Guiding the current movement to implement evidence-based practice with young children with disabilities are a number of questions asking: Which interventions or practices are most effective for young children with special needs? Under what conditions, by whom, and for whom should they be implemented to make a measurable and meaningful impact on the lives of young children? What level of evidence is needed to determine that a practice or intervention is effective? How does the field of early childhood support the dissemination of evidence-based practice? How can early educators and interventionists access information about evidence-based practices? (e.g., Guralnick, 1997; Odom & Wolery, 2003; Shonkoff, 2000). The process of deciding what constitutes the evidence behind evidence-based practice and how to actually put evidence-based practices into practice that improves the outcomes of young children presents some of the most salient challenges to the field of early childhood.

To better understand what evidence-based practice in early childhood entails, a brief discussion of the terminology related to evidence-based practice in early childhood special education is provided along with information about the criteria proposed for determining what constitutes evidence. Examples of practices that are representative of the best available evidence in early childhood education and intervention are provided along with suggestions for how educators, policymakers and others might currently access evidence-based practices for early education and intervention.

DEFINING EVIDENCE-BASED PRACTICE

Most professionals providing education and intervention to young children with disabilities would agree that using intervention practices supported by research is important. However, there is not general agreement as to the definition of evidence-based practice or necessarily what constitutes the evidence behind evidence-based intervention or practices (e.g., Cook, Tankersley, & Landrum, 2009; Kazdin, 2008; Odom et al., 2005; Slavin, 2008; Snyder, 2006). Although review syntheses concerning research evidence were increasingly available, Dunst, Trivette, and Cutspec (2002) realized that without a working definition of evidence-based practice, the utility of such information by early educators and interventionists in practice would be limited. Indeed, the lack of consensus as to what is meant by the term evidence-based practice, or how to identify evidence-based intervention practices from the myriad of practices available, ultimately impedes their dissemination and use. Early educators and interventionists are at a disadvantage in terms of being able to access and utilize information about intervention practices most likely to result in desired outcomes if the criteria for what constitutes evidence is unclear.

Evidence-based practice encompasses more broadly the process and methods used for making informed decisions regarding intervention, teaching, and learning approaches (see Buysse & Wesley, 2006; Carta & Kong, 2007; Snyder, 2006). A number of definitions for evidence-based practice and outcomes in early childhood intervention have been proposed (e.g., Buysse and Wesley, 2006; Dunst & Trivette, 2009; McWilliam, Wolery, & Odom, 2001; Snyder, 2006) and for the most part, all refer to evidence-based practice as an approach to intervention, and not only to specific practices or interventions that have a scientific, empirical, or research base. Aligned with definitions of evidence-based practice adopted by other fields, including medicine (Sackett, Rosenberg, Muir Gray, Haynes, & Richardson, 2000), clinical psychology (Kazdin, 2008), school psychology (Kratochwill & Stoiber, 2002), communication disorders (ASHA, 2005) and general education (Slavin, 2008), Snyder (2006) refers to evidence-based practice in early intervention as "a process for making informed decisions that involves considering not only the best available research evidence about certain treatments or practices but also knowledge gained through experience and values" (p. 39). Central to the definitions embraced by these and other fields, and generally included in those proposed for EI/ECSE, is that evidence-based practice encompasses an approach that considers research or scientific evidence in addition to professional as well as family experience, knowledge, and values in making decisions about how best to meet the needs of children and families (Buysse & Wesley, 2006 p. 12; Snyder, 2006). When speaking more broadly in terms of an evidence-based practice approach, there are aspects of assessment and measurement of the fidelity of intervention delivery, reliability of measurement, monitoring of progress and outcomes, and professional development activities that are integral components of an evidence-based practice approach (e.g., Carta, 2002; McConnell, 2000).

In the wake of the Education Sciences Reform Act of 2002, the U.S. Department of Education established the Institute of Education Sciences (IES) (http://ies.ed.gov) as the research arm of the department. The mission of the IES through four centers, one of which is the National Center for Special Education Research, as described on their Web site, is to provide national leadership in expanding the knowledge and understanding of education to provide educators, researchers, policy makers, parents, and the public with reliable information about the condition and progress of education. The IES works toward this goal in part by supporting research grants and promoting the use, development, and application of knowledge gained from research evaluated through the What Works Clearinghouse (WWC; http://www.whatworks.ed.gov).

The WWC was designed to review, evaluate, and disseminate rigorous and relevant research and evaluation to educators and others by providing a central source of scientific evidence in education. Through the WWC, intervention reports within specific topic areas, which are rated based on WWC evidence standards, are generated and made available on the WWC Web site. Ratings of interventions conducted through a strategic review process range from "positive," "mixed effects," to "no discernible effects," or "negative." Eligibility screens are conducted to determine whether studies meet evidence standards (e.g., by providing strong evidence, weaker evidence, or insufficient evidence).

Presently, the WWC considers well-designed and well-implemented randomized controlled trials (RCTs) as providing the strongest evidence, while quasi-experimental designs were considered to provide weak evidence or only to meet standards with reservations. Recent papers outlining the evidence standards for regression discontinuity (Schochet et al., 2010) and single-case designs (Kratochwill et al., 2010) have been released and are available on the WWC Web site (http://www.whatworks.ed.gov). Standards for these research designs are provided that may result in the WWC broadening the criteria used to include designs other than RCTs in its database. This is particularly important for research conducted with children with special needs given the smaller sample sizes and heterogeneous characteristics of children with disabilities, making it almost impossible to use research methodology that requires large numbers of participants (Collins & Salzberg, 2005; Dunst et al., 2002; Odom et al., 2005; Snyder, 2006).

Evidence evaluated through the WWC is synthesized into report formats providing summary information as to whether the extent of the evidence was small, medium, or large. From these reports, users can compare ratings of effectiveness across studies. The WWC provides practitioners and policy makers with assessments about the quality of the research evidence, and based on reviews of research as well as the opinions and experiences of nationally recognized expert panel members, practice guides containing recommendations for educators are available to users. Although IES and the WWC includes early childhood and early childhood special education as areas of inquiry and importance for the WWC, to date, very few research syntheses are available for early childhood, which at this time is limited to preschool-aged children between ages 3 and 5 years in the WWC database. This is seen as a missed opportunity to provide summative information in the area of early childhood related to evidence-based interventions.

EXAMPLES FROM RELATED FIELDS

Health Care

Associated fields have approached the process of identifying and disseminating their approach to evidence-based practice in a number of ways that have been informative to the field of early intervention—or could be. For instance, the medical field, in particular through the work of the Cochrane Collaboration, provides summaries of studies across the health care field (Volmink, Siegried, Robertson, & Gulmezoglu, 2004). Each review addresses a specific question related to health care, policy, or methodology and includes research on a topic that meets certain criteria as to whether or not there is conclusive evidence about a specific treatment. An online advisor from the American Medical Association (JAMAevidence) also provides users with tools for understanding and applying the medical literature and for making clinical and diagnostic decisions. The Web site offers users tools to learn how to recognize and ask questions about clinical applications, gather evidence from the literature, check the best available evidence for indicators of validity, importance, and usefulness, and to interpret the applicability of the evidence to specific problems given patient preferences and values (http://jamaevidence.com).

School Psychology

In school psychology, a number of resources have been developed to evaluate the level of evidence in support of interventions, including an edition of the journal of the Division of School Psychology, *School Psychology Quarterly*, in 2002, and a portion of their Web site for the National Association of School Psychology. Work described by Kratochwill and Stoiber (2002), supported in part through the American Psychological Association, chronicles the process of constructing a knowledge base of school psychology research with the purpose of providing consumers the opportunity to draw their own conclusions based on the evidence provided. Information ranges from content about school- and community-based intervention programs for social and behavioral problems, and academic intervention programs, to family and parent intervention and methodological issues including single-subject research designs and group designs. Criteria for coding research included designating treatments as "well-established," "promising interventions," or "treatments widely practice with only limited support." Interventions were coded on dimensions ranging from having at least two good studies demonstrating efficacy through an experimental-control group design or a series of single-case studies. Practice guidelines to facilitate the adoption of evidence-based practices by trainers and practitioners and to yield functional scientific information for psychology and education have also been designed (Kratochwill & Shernoff, 2004; White & Kratochwill, 2005) to facilitate the dissemination of the information.

THE ROLE OF PROFESSIONAL ORGANIZATIONS AND JOURNALS IN DEFINING EVIDENCE-BASED PRACTICE

The Council for Exceptional Children (CEC) is an international professional organization dedicated to improving the educational success of individuals with disabilities (http://www.cec.sped.org). CEC advocates for appropriate governmental policies, sets professional standards, and provides professional development through scholarly professional journals, conferences, and resource materials. The CEC describes evidence-based special education practice as a strategy or intervention designed for use by special educators and intended to support the education of individuals with exceptional learning needs. Through the CEC Professional Standards and Practice Committee, the CEC has proposed criteria for distinguishing the methodological levels of evidence-based practice recommendations (CEC, 2006). Methodological quality indicators published in a special issue of the journal *Exceptional Children* (2005) were used as the basis upon which to develop rubrics for coding of studies that special educators might use to support the education of exceptional children. The proposed criteria included research-based, promising, and emerging practices. Methodological criteria ranging from levels of experimental, correlational, or qualitative studies are outlined along with associated practice recommendations. The CEC publishes a number of journals for researchers and practitioners on current research findings and curricular activities that are useful for informing research and practice (e.g., the *Journal of Special Education and Teaching Exceptional Children*).

The Division for Early Childhood of the Council for Exceptional Children (DEC) is an international organization promoting policies and advances in evidence-based practices for children birth through 8 years of age with disabilities and other special needs, their families, and professionals. The DEC generally defines evidence-based practices as the integration of best available research with professional and family wisdom and experience. The DEC Task Force on Recommended Practices originally published a set of recommended practices in 1993 that has been updated (Sandall, Hemmeter, Smith, & McLean, 2005) to provide guidance on effective practices for improving the development and learning outcomes of young children with disabilities and their families. Using a process that included the examination of the best available research evidence from over 1,000 articles from journals relevant to EI/ECSE and a process of professional and field validation that included focus groups of stakeholders including practitioners, researchers, and administrators as well as family members, national survey respondents, and hundreds of reviewers, the present DEC Recommended Practices guide includes 240 recommended practices organized under topical strand areas covering child-focused interventions, family-based topics, policies, procedures, and systems change, assessment, personnel preparation, technology applications, and interdisciplinary models. The criteria used to determine the inclusion of articles was that they had to be original research that involved children birth through 5 years with disabilities, their families, or personnel, as well as policies and systems change procedures that support effective practice. Articles were evaluated for evidence using criteria that related specifically to the type of design employed (e.g., qualitative, single-subject, random assignment) and included review of the research design, sample, setting, outcome measures, intervention duration, fidelity, findings, and the recommended practice(s) supported by the study. The criteria by which they were selected included evaluation as to the theoretical base, methodological integrity, consensus, reliability, and social validity (Smith, McLean, Sandall, Snyder, & Ramsey, 2005). There are now a number of resource materials that support the DEC Recommended Practices guide designed for early educators and interventionists, including a program assessment guide (Hemmeter, Joseph, Smith, & Sandall, 2001), a videotape illustrating the practices, a personnel preparation guide (Stayton, Miller, & Dinnebeil, 2002) links to research-based practitioner-oriented articles at http://www.dec -sped.org, and a workbook for assessing use of the recommended practices (Hemmeter, Smith, Sandall, & Askew, 2005). Journals published through the DEC that cover topics related to young children with disabilities include the *Journal of Early Intervention, Young Exceptional Children*, and the *Young Exceptional Children Monographs*.

The DEC Recommended Practices guide (Sandall et al., 2005) was derived as described from an extensive synthesis of research and experience-based knowledge of the EI/ECSE literature between 1990 and 1998 (Smith et al., 2002). The guidelines, while comprehensive, have differential levels of empirical support given the state of the literature during the review period conducted over a decade ago. They are valuable in that they represent collective wisdom of the field about practices that have been found to be useful, if not effective, for some children. The collection provides a framework for defining quality practices associated to positive outcomes and serve as a resource to help inform the evidence-based practice decisions of educators and interventionists (Snyder, 2006). Research on the use of the recommended practices, however, suggests that like other similar resources, they are not necessarily routinely embedded into personnel preparation programs (e.g., Bruder & Dunst, 2005) or used systematically by practitioners (e.g., McLean, Snyder, Smith, & Sandall, 2002). There continues to be a failure in the field to translate research into practice. Bruder (2010) suggests a number of reasons for these translational research failures, including reliance on process rather than child and family intervention outcomes and a systematic and reliable process for identifying and utilizing evidence-based practices, among other systemic constraints related to professional development.

WHAT COUNTS AS EVIDENCE?

Perhaps the most complex issue facing the evidence-based practice movement, and certainly the thorniest, has been the question of what is considered to be evidence supporting a practice or intervention as evidence-based. Odom et al. (2005) mused that while there was generally widespread agreement that early intervention and education practices should be guided by research, "the devil is in the details" (p. 137). Questions related to whether studies of early intervention practices are sufficiently rigorous, specifically: (1) How many studies or replications are needed? (2) How large an effect is necessary to indicate meaningful change? (3) What format is needed to disseminate information that will be usable by those delivering intervention? These are all questions that, as yet, are undecided (e.g., Cook, Tankersley, & Landrum, 2009; Snyder, 2006). With these important questions about what constitutes evidence-based practices left essentially to interpretation, what has occurred is an overuse of the term evidence-based and, to some extent, a dilution of the evidence that does exit and would be beneficial to inform intervention practice.

The process of distilling which practices have sufficient evidence supporting them and which do not requires some agreement about the methodology used to test their effectiveness. This is perhaps the biggest deterrent to the identification of evidence-based practices in

EI/ECSE. It is generally understood that different research methodologies should be used to address the effectiveness of interventions and specific practices (e.g., Huston, 2008; National Research Council and Institute of Medicine, 2000; Snyder, 2006); as multiple sources of evidence may produce converging evidence about effective practices (Dunst et al., 2002). Unfortunately, however, the acceptance of findings from studies using other than randomized trials to support their use continues to be minimal (Dunst et al. 2002; Kratochwill et al., 2010; Odom et al., 2005). Research findings that weighed most heavily as having the biggest impact on policy initiatives, for example, have been research based on high-quality methodology, including random assignment and longitudinal studies that are replicated (Huston, 2008). While admittedly there is a lot of research in early intervention that has not been conducted under ideal circumstances (e.g., Odom et al., 2005), the field has benefitted from a rich history of blended instructional methodology, some of high quality, some less so, but from which early educators and interventionists have drawn in their treatment of infants, toddlers, and young children with disabilities (Odom & Wolery, 2003). The field will be seriously disadvantaged if instead of continuing to draw upon the research in early childhood that does have adequate evidence as identified using a broad array of appropriate methodology, it instead becomes mired in "nitpicking the limits of existing research" (McCall, 2009, p. 3).

It could be argued that to some extent, this has already been the case. As of yet, early childhood special education, and in general the special education field, does not have agreed-upon guidelines for determining whether a practice or intervention is evidence-based or even effective (Odom et al., 2005). Several approaches have been proposed, including ranking levels of evidence for rigor (Dunst et al., 2002; Dunst & Trivette, 2009; Snyder, 2006) or using stages or standards of evidence (see Groark & McCall, 2008; Odom et al., 2005). While these have some merit for helping to provide an organizational framework for considering the various methodological options, they have been criticized for being misguided because "different kinds of efficacy questions demand the use of different kinds of research methodologies" (Dunst et al., 2002, p. 2). Others suggest that in applying levels of evidence, one need not designate specific levels of evidence as being superior to others; rather, that they permit different levels of inference (Snyder, 2006). Quality indicators are another method proposed for evaluating the contributions of different methodologies (e.g., CEC, 2006; Snyder, 2006; WWC), including group or single-subject experimental designs and correlational, qualitative, and evaluation research. In these systems, the evidence base is ranked using criteria that specifies whether a practice or intervention has a certain number of high-quality studies to support the practice and intervention effect sizes that meet a certain criteria (CEC, 2006; Kratochwill et al., 2010).

In isolation, the research literature does not inform practitioners about which practices will most likely benefit the heterogeneous children and families they serve when implemented under real-world conditions. Nor does it advise how to maintain intervention fidelity when the individualization of interventions is by definition what early interventionists do. "More rigorous research on the 'what'—the intervention-will not tell us 'how' to implement with fidelity and good outcomes over time and across practitioners in complex settings" (Blase, Van Dyke, & Fixsen, 2009, p. 14). How to monitor progress to ensure that children are making expected outcomes, or how to make alterations in intervention protocol to meet individual needs of children, are intervention decisions that require knowledge and experience as well as access to evidence-based practice techniques. McCall (2009) points out that "the simple dissemination of research information is not likely to be sufficient to prescribe what should be done in practice" (p. 7). An evidence-based practice approach encompasses not only the identification of interventions and practices with rigorous research evidence supporting their use, but also the means to translate that evidence into actual practice.

USING THE BEST EVIDENCE AVAILABLE TO INFORM PRACTICE WITH YOUNG CHILDREN

Determining the best fit between practices and the needs of a family or child requires making decisions about how convincing the evidence is in supporting the practice(s) and whether the practices will be implemented within the given context (Cook et al., 2009). Not all interventions will be effective or necessarily appropriate for all children and families under all conditions. While some interventions and practices will be effective for certain children or families under specific conditions, those same practices may not lead to desired outcomes with children and families who have different needs, or by different parents or teachers with divergent interaction or teaching styles (Cook, et al., 2009; Forness, Kavale, Blum, & Lloyd, 1997). The intervention practices evaluated and recommended by the What Works Clearinghouse and the DEC Recommended Practices, through professional organizations (e.g., the American Speech-Language-Hearing Association [ASHA] and the Council for Exceptional Children [CEC]), and technical assistance projects (e.g., NECTAC) provide information that requires skilled users to assemble and translate into intervention practices that can be used and assimilated in practice. These resources constitute what can be considered the best available evidence for use within an evidence-based practice approach.

Using the general strand headings from the DEC Recommended Practices (Sandall et al. 2005), what follows are examples of some recent innovations in early childhood special education for which there is some level of evidence. This summary is only for illustrative purposes about information that may be useful in applications of evidence-based practice and in no way attempts to be inclusive of all practices described in the DEC Recommended Practices guide, the WWC Web site, or from other evidence-based practice resources. Please refer to the WWC, the DEC Recommended Practices guide (Sandall et al., 2005); the National Early Childhood Technical Assistance Center (NECTAC, http://www .nectac.org); the National Association for the Education of Young Children (NAEYC, http://www.naeyc.org); the Center on the Developing Child at Harvard University (http://www.developingchild.harvard .edu); and the National Dissemination Center for Children with Disabilities (NICHCY, http://www.nichcy.org) for more resources related to evidence-based intervention and practices for young children with disabilities.

ASSESSMENT IN EARLY CHILDHOOD

In general, assessment should provide useful information for purposes of screening, diagnosis, guiding intervention and instruction, and for providing information about program effectiveness and impact (National Research Council, 2008; Neisworth & Bagnato, 2005). Assessment should provide meaningful and useful information about infants, toddlers, and young children with disabilities, the environments in which they live and learn, and about their interactions with others. Input from multiple sources, including parents and professionals, and through direct observation, provides the most valuable and comprehensive information upon which to base intervention decision making (Sandall et al., 2005).

Response to Intervention (RtI)

RtI is an approach that integrates identification, assessment and intervention in a problem-solving approach that has been used extensively for school-aged children (Fuchs & Fuchs, 2006) but more recently utilized to inform intervention for young children (e.g., Buzhardt et al., 2010; Coleman, Buysse, & Neitzel, 2006; Fox, Carta, Strain, Dunlap, & Hemmeter, 2009; Greenwood et al., 2008; Koutsoftas, Harmon, & Gray, 2009; VanDerHeyden, Snyder, Broussard, & Ramsdell, 2010). The RtI approach builds on traditional early intervention practice because it gives providers systematic procedures for deciding when a child may not be making expected progress, when a child is responding to intervention, and when to change or modify an intervention. See also the Center for RtI in Early Childhood (CRTIEC, http://www.crtiec.org/index.shtml); the RtI Action Network (http://www.rtinetwork.org/learn/rti-in-pre-kindergarten); and the Center on Social Emotional Intervention for Young Children (http://www.challengingbehavior.org).

Progress-Monitoring Measures

One format used for measuring the progress of young children, known as Individual Growth and Development Indicators (IGDIs; Carta, Greenwood, Walker, & Buzhardt, 2010), has been used successfully to screen, monitor progress, and inform intervention within a decision-making format, including an RtI approach for infants and young children for communication and early literacy (Greenwood et al., 2008; McConnell & Missall, 2008). Developed as an alternative to traditional measures to provide practitioners with an authentic, technically adequate, sensitive, and efficient measure that can be used to generate individual child- and program-level information and that informs intervention (see also http://www.igdi.ku.edu). Customized dynamic reports of child progress, interventions used, staff, and child data including individual growth charts are available to users to facilitate progress monitoring. Published reports documenting the technical adequacy of the IGDIs are available (e.g., Greenwood, Carta, Walker, Hughes, & Weathers, 2006; Greenwood & Walker, 2010).

CHILD-FOCUSED INTERVENTIONS

Child-focused practices and interventions designed to improve the outcomes of young children encompass a large number of the interventions described in the literature. Such practices guide how young children are taught, how practices or strategies are implemented, and how their performance is monitored (Wolery, 2005). The main strategies covered under this intervention strand include adults purposefully designing environments to promote children's active engagement, learning, and to influence children's participation and experiences.

Naturalistic Language Strategies

Decades of rigorous single-subject and group research on naturalistic approaches to early communication and language intervention with young children including Milieu Teaching (e.g., Kaiser, Hancock, & Nietfeld, 2000), Prelinguistic Milieu Teaching (e.g., Yoder & Stone, 2006), and Responsive Interaction (e.g.,Warren, Fey, Finestack, Brady, Bredin-Oja, & Fleming, 2008;Yoder & Warren, 2001) provide the foundation for naturalistic communication interventions. These strategies are designed particularly for use in the context of the everyday interactions between parents, caregivers and children (e.g., Walker, Bigelow, & Harjusola-Webb, 2008).

Dialogic Reading

Dialogic reading (e.g., Dale, Crain-Thoreson, Notari-Syverson, & Cole, 1996, Justice & Pullen, 2003; Whitehurst, Arnold, Epstein, & Angell, 1994), an interactive shared picture-book reading intervention that uses milieu and responsive interaction strategies to improve early literacy skills, expressive vocabulary, and narrative skills, was recently listed by the WWC as a practice that produced positive outcomes in oral language skills (WWC, 2010).

PERSONNEL PREPARATION

The preparation and skill level of those who deliver intervention to young children with disabilities can have a significant impact on the outcomes of the children and families receiving services (Tout, Zaslow, & Berry, 2006). Interventionists and special educators who deliver services to young children and their families may work directly providing services to children, or may provide services in consultation with other special educators, parents, or both (Buysse & Wesley, 2006). Personnel preparation also directly impacts the training of students in higher education to be educators and interventionists at the preservice and consultation level (e.g., Wesley, Buysse, & Keyes, 2000). As described by Buysse, Winton, and Rous (2009), what constitutes professional development can vary greatly, from attendance at a workshop to an entire semester-long course, with as much variability in between. Campbell and Sawyer (2009) analyzed participants' summative statements about their professional development and recommended practices for service delivery, finding that services were more often related to beliefs than professional development levels. Another study found that level of expertise impacted home visiting outcomes when services were delivered by trained nurses rather than paraprofessionals (e.g., Olds et al., 2004; Center on the Developing Child, 2007).

ON BECOMING AN EVIDENCE-BASED PRACTICE

As a field, early intervention/early childhood special education is in the process of embracing evidence-based practice as a paradigm for intervention service delivery. Knowledge about effective practices and how to use the best available evidence to guide intervention decision making will continue to be generated and contribute to improving the quality of the early intervention that young children and their families receive. Understanding how to interpret and assimilate that information into practice is one of our next challenges. The questions asked at the beginning of this chapter will no doubt continue to guide these efforts. We will continue to explore how to identify those intervention and assessment practices that are most effective for young children and their families and to distill the conditions under which those practices will have the largest impact. As a field, we understand that this process will need to be individualized, adding to the complexity of identifying those practices that are most effective and that help to inform evidence-based practice. It is important, however, that we move forward with becoming an evidence-based field in a thoughtful way. Blase, Van Dyke, and Fixsen (2009) caution that "Understanding the contributions and limitations of rigorous intervention research relative to implementation is critical. Scientific rigor is important. Choosing well is important. Implementation is hard work" (p. 14). They remind us that simply identifying the "what" from more rigorous research will not tell us "how" to implement practices with good fidelity or guarantee good outcomes. As we proceed, we will need to make sure that we both install and then support the processes needed to sustain the implementation of evidence-based practice across the complex conditions under which early intervention services are delivered.

References

American Speech-Language-Hearing Association (ASHA). (2005). *Evidence-based practice in communication disorders* [position statement]. Retrieved from http://www.asha.org/policy

Blase, K. A., Van Dyke, M., & Fixsen, D. (2009). Evidence-based programming in the context of practice and policy. *Social Policy Report, 23*(3). Society for Research in Child Development.

Bruder, M. B. (2010). Early childhood intervention: A promise to children and families for their future. *Exceptional Children, 76*(3), 339–355.

Bruder, M. B., & Dunst, C. (2005). Personnel preparation in recommended early intervention practices: Degree of emphasis across disciplines. *Topics in Early Childhood Special Education, 25*, 25–33.

Buysse, V., & Wesley, P. W. (2006). Evidence-based practice: How did it emerge and what does it really mean for the early childhood field? In V. Buysse & P. Wesley (Eds.), *Evidence-based practice in the early childhood field* (pp. 1–34). Washington, DC: Zero to Three Press.

Buysse, V., Winton, P., & Rous, B. (2009). Reaching consensus on a definition of professional development for the early childhood field. *Topics in Early Childhood Special Education, 28*, 235–243.

Buzhardt, J., Greenwood, C., Walker, D., Carta, J., Terry, B., & Garrett, M. (2010). A web-based tool to support data-based early intervention decision making. *Topics in Early Childhood Special Education, 29*, 201–213.

Campbell, P. H., & Sawyer, L. B. (2009). Changing early intervention providers' home visiting skills through participation in professional development. *Topics in Early Childhood Special Education, 28*, 219–234.

Carta, J. J. (2002). An early childhood special education research agenda in a culture of accountability for results. *Journal of Early Intervention, 25*(2), 102–104.

Carta, J. J., Greenwood, C. R., Walker, D., & Buzhardt, J. (2010). *Using IGDIs: Monitoring progress and improving intervention results for infants and young children.* Baltimore: Paul H. Brookes.

Carta, J. J., & Kong, N. Y. (2007). Trends and issues in interventions for preschoolers with developmental disabilities. In S. L. Odom, R. H. Horner, M. E. Snell, & J. Blancher (Eds.) *Handbook of developmental disabilities* (pp. 181–198). New York: Guilford Press.

Center on the Developing Child at Harvard University. (2007). *A science-based framework for early childhood policy: Using evidence to improve outcomes in learning, behavior, and health for vulnerable children.* Retrieved from http://www.developingchild.harvard.edu

Cochran Collaboration. (n.d.) Retrieved from http://www.cochrane.org

Coleman, M. R., Buysse, V., & Neitzel, J. (2006). *Recognition and response: An early intervening system for young children at risk for learning disabilities. Full report.* Chapel Hill: University of North Carolina, FPG Child Development Institute.

Collins, S., & Salzberg, C. (2005). Scientifically based research and students with severe disabilities: Where do educators find evidence-based practices? *Rural Special Education Quarterly, 24*, 60–63.

Cook, B. G., Tankersley, M., & Landrum, T. J. (2009). Determining evidence-based practices in special education. *Exceptional Children, 75*(3), 365–383.

Council for Exceptional Children. (n.d.) *CEC Today, Evidence-based practice—wanted, needed, and hard to get.* Retrieved from http://www.cec.sped.org

Dale, P. S., Crain-Thoreson, C., Notari-Syverson, A., & Cole, K. (1996). Parent-child book reading as an intervention technique for young children with language delays. *Topics in Early Childhood Special Education, 16*, 213–235.

Division for Early Childhood (DEC). (2006, October). *Research priorities for early intervention and early childhood special education.* Author.

Dunst, C. J., & Trivette, C. M. (2009). Using research evidence to inform and evaluate early childhood intervention practices. *Topics in Early Childhood Special Education, 29*, 40–52.

Dunst, C., Trivette, C., & Cutspec, P. (2002). *Toward an operational definition of evidence-based practice.* Retrieved from http://www.nasddds.org/pdf/TowardAnOperationalDefinition.pdf

Education Sciences Reform Act of 2002, Pub. L. 107-229, Title I-B, 20 U.S.C. §§ 9533, 9562.

Forness, S. R., Kavale, K. A., Blum, I. M., & Lloyd, J. W. (1997). What works in special education and related services: Using meta-analysis to guide practice. *Teaching Exceptional Children, 29*, 4–9.

Fox, L., Carta, J., Strain, P., Dunlap, G., & Hemmeter, M. L. (2009). Response to intervention and the Pyramid Model. Tampa, FL: University of South Florida, Technical Assistance Center on Social Emotional Intervention for Young Children.

Fuchs, D., & Fuchs, L. S. (2006). Introduction to responsiveness-to-intervention: What, why and how valid is it? *Reading Research Quarterly, 41*, 92–99.

Greenwood, C. R., Carta, J. J., Baggett, K., Buzhardt, J., Walker, D., & Terry, B. (2008). Best practices in integrating progress monitoring and response-to-intervention concepts into early childhood systems. In A. Thomas & J. Grimes (Eds.), *Best Practices in School Psychology* (pp. 535–547). Bethesda, MD: National Association of School Psychologists.

Greenwood, C. R., Carta, J. J., Walker, D., Hughes, K., & Weathers, M. (2006). Preliminary investigations of the application of the Early Communication Indicator (ECI) for infants and toddlers. *Journal of Early Intervention, 28*, 178–196.

Greenwood, C., & Walker, D. (2010). Development and validation of IGDIs. In J. J. Carta, C. Greenwood, D. Walker, & J. Buzhardt, *Using IGDIs: Monitoring progress and improving intervention results for infants and young children* (pp. 145–177). Baltimore, MD: Paul H. Brookes.

Groark, C. J., & McCall, R. B. (2008). Community-based interventions and services. In M. Rutter, D. Bishop, D. Pine, S. Scott, J. Stevenson, E. Taylor, & A. Thapar (Eds.), *Rutter's child and adolescent psychiatry* (5th ed., pp. 971–988). London: Blackwell Publishing.

Guralnick, M. J. (1997). *The effectiveness of early intervention.* Baltimore: Paul H. Brookes.

Guralnick, M. J. (2005). Early intervention for children with intellectual disabilities: Current knowledge and future prospects. *Journal of Applied Research in Intellectual Disabilities, 18*, 313–324.

Harbin, G., Rous, B., & McLean, M. (2005). Issues in designing state accountability systems. *Journal of Early Intervention, 27*, 137–164.

Head Start Act of 1998. Pub. L. 97-35, 42 W.S.C §§9801, et seq. Retrieved from http://eclkc.ohs.acf.hhs.gov/hslc/Head%20Start%20Program/Program %20Design%20and%20Management/Head%20Start%20Requirements/Heas %20Start%20Act/headstartact.html

Hebbeler, K., Barton, L. R., & Mallik, S. (2008). Assessment and accountability for programs serving young children with disabilities. *Exceptionality, 16*, 2–18.

Hemmeter, M. L., Joseph, G., Smith, B. J., & Sandall, S. (Eds.). (2001). *DEC recommended practices program assessment: Improving practices for young children with special needs and their families.* Missoula, MT: Division for Early Childhood.

Hemmeter, M. L., Smith, B. J., Sandall, S., & Askew, L. (Eds.). (2005) *DEC recommended practices workbook: Improving practices for young children with special needs and their families.* Missoula, MT: Division for Early Childhood.

Huston, A. C. (2008). From research to policy and back. *Child Development, 79*, 1–12.

Individuals with Disabilities Education Improvement Act of 2004, Pub. L. 108-446.

Justice, L. M., & Pullen, P. C. (2003). Promising interventions for promoting emergent literacy skills: Three evidence-based approaches. *Topics in Early Childhood Special Education, 23*, 99–113.

Kaiser, A. P., Hancock, T. B., & Nietfeld, J. P. (2000). The effects of parent-implemented enhanced milieu teaching on the social communication of children who have autism. *Journal of Early Education and Development, 4*, 423–446

Kazdin, A. E. (2008). Evidence-based treatment and practice: New opportunities to bridge clinical research and practice, enhance the knowledge base, and improve patient care. *American Psychologist, 63*(3), 146–159.

Koutsoftas, A. D., Harmon, M. T., & Gray, S. (2009). The effect of tier 2 intervention for phonemic awareness in a response-to-intervention model in low-income preschool classrooms. *Language, Speech, and Hearing Services in Schools, 40*, 116–130.

Kratochwill, T. R., Hitchcock, J., Horner, R. H., Levin, J. R., Odom, S. L., Rindskopf, D. M., & Shadish, W. R. (2010). Single-case designs technical documentation. Retrieved from What Works Clearinghouse, http://ies.ed.gov/ncee/wwc/ pdf/wwc_scd.pdf

Kratochwill, T. R., & Shernoff, E. S. (2004). Evidence-based practice: Promoting evidence-based interventions in school psychology. *School Psychology Review, 33*, 34–48.

Kratochwill, T. R., & Stoiber, K. C. (2002). Evidence-based interventions in school psychology: Conceptual foundations of the Procedural and Coding Manual of Division 16 and the Society for the Study of School Psychology Task Force. *School Psychology Quarterly, 17*, 341–389.

Lazar, I., Darlington, R., Murray, H., Royce, J., & Snipper, A. (1982). Lasting effects of early education: A report from the Consortium for Longitudinal Studies. *Monographs of the Society for Research in Child Development, 47*(2–3, Serial No. 195).

McCall, R. B. (2009). Evidence-based programming in the context of practice and policy. *Social Policy Report, 23*(3). Society for Research in Child Development.

McConnell, S. R. (2000). Assessment in early intervention and early childhood special education: Building on the past to project into our future. *Topics in Early Childhood Special Education, 20*, 43–48.

McConnell, S. R., & Missall, K. N. (2008). Best practices in monitoring progress for preschool children. In A. Thomas & J. Grimes (Eds.), *Best practices in school psychology* (5th ed., pp. 561–573). Washington, DC: National Association of School Psychologists.

McLean, M., Snyder, P., Smith, B. J., & Sandall, S. (2002). The DEC recommended practices in early intervention/early childhood special education: Social validation. Journal of Early Intervention, *25*, 120–128.

McWilliam, R. A., Wolery, M., & Odom, S. L. (2001). Instructional perspectives in inclusive preschool classrooms. In M. J. Guralnick (Ed.), *Early childhood inclusion: Focus on change* (pp. 503–527). Baltimore: Paul H. Brookes.

National Research Council. (2008). *Early Childhood Assessment: Why, What, and How.* Committee on Developmental Outcomes and Assessments for Young Children (C. E. Snow & S. B. Van Hemel, Eds.). Board on Children, Youth, and Families, Board on Testing and Assessment, Division of Behavioral and Social Sciences and Education. Washington, DC: National Academies Press.

National Research Council and Institute of Medicine. (2000). *From neurons to neighborhoods: The science of early childhood development.* Committee on Integrating the Science of Early Childhood Development. J. P. Shonkoff & D. A. Phillips (Eds.). Board on Children, Youth and Families, Commission on Behavioral and Social Sciences and Education. Washington, DC: National Academy Press.

No Child Left Behind Act of 2001, Pub. L. 107-110, 115 Stat. 1425.

Odom, S. L., Brantlinger, E., Gersten, R., Horner, R. H., Thompson, B., & Harris, K. R. (2005). Research in special education: Scientific methods and evidence-based practices. *Exceptional Children, 71*(2), 137–149.

Odom. S. L., & Wolery, M. (2003). A unified theory of practice in early intervention/early childhood special education: Evidence-based practices. *Journal of Special Education, 37*, 164–173.

Office of Management and Budget (OMB). (2006). Program assessment: IDEA Special Education Grants for Infants and Families. Retrieved from http://www.whitehouse.gov/omb/expectmore

Olds, D. L., Robinson, J. A., Pettit, L., Luckey, D. W., Holmburg, J., Ng, R. K., et al. (2004). Effects of home visits by paraprofessionals and by nurses: Age 4 follow-up results of a randomized trial, *Pediatrics, 114*(6), 1560–1568.

Ramey, C. T., & Campbell, F. A. (1992). Poverty, early childhood education, and academic competence: The abecedarian experiment. In A. Huston (Ed.), *Children in Poverty.* New York: Cambridge University Press.

Sackett, D. L., Rosenberg, W. M. C., Muir Gray, J. A., Haynes, R. B., & Richardson, W. S. (1996). *British Medical Journal, 312*, 71–72.

Sandall, S., Hemmeter, M. L., Smith, B. J., & McLean, M. E. (Eds.). (2005) *DEC recommended practices: A comprehensive guide for practical application in early intervention/early childhood special education.* Missoula, MT: Division for Early Childhood.

Schochet, P., Cook, T., Deke, J., Imbens, G., Lockwood, J. R., Porter, J., & Smith, J. (2010). Standards for regression discontinuity designs. Retrieved from What Works Clearinghouse, http://ies.ed.gov/ncee/wwc/pdf/wwc_rd.pdf

Senate Committee on Governmental Affairs. (1993). Government Performance and Results Act of 1993 Report (No. 103-58).

Shonkoff, J. P. (2000). Science, policy, and practice: Three cultures in search of a shared mission. *Child Development, 71*, 181–187.

Shonkoff, J. P., & Meisels, S. J. (2000). *Handbook of early intervention* (2nd ed.). New York: Cambridge University Press.

Slavin, R. E. (2008). Perspectives on evidence-based research in education: What works? Issues in synthesizing educational program evaluations. *Educational Researcher, 37*(1), 5–14.

Smith, B. J., McLean, M. E., Sandall, S., Snyder, P., & Ramsey, A. B. (2005). DEC recommended practices: The procedures and evidence base used to establish them. In S. Sandall, M. L. Hemmeter, B. J. Smith, & M. E. McLean (Eds.), *DEC recommended practices: A comprehensive guide for practical application in early intervention/early childhood special education* (pp. 27–39). Longmont, CO: Sopris West.

Smith, B. J., Strain, P. S., Snyder, P., Sandall, S., McLean, M. E., Ramsey A. B., & Sumi, W. C. (2002). DEC recommended practices: A review of nine years of EI/ECSE research literature. *Journal of Early Intervention, 25*(2), 108–119.

Snyder, P. (2006). Best available research evidence: Impact on research in early childhood. In V. Buysse & P. Wesley (Eds.), *Evidence-based practice in the early childhood field* (pp. 35–70). Washington, DC: Zero to Three Press.

Stayton, F. D., Miller, P. S., & Dinnebeil, L. A. (Eds.) (2002) *Personnel preparation in early childhood special education: implementing the DEC recommended practices.* Missoula, MT: Division for Early Childhood.

Tout, K., Zaslow, M., & Berry, D. (2006). Quality and Qualifications. In M. Zaslow & I. Martinez-Beck (Eds.), *Critical issues in early childhood professional development* (pp. 77–110). Baltimore: Paul H. Brookes.

VanDerHeyden, A. M., Snyder, P. A., Broussard, C., & Ramsdell, K. (2010). Measuring response to early literacy intervention with preschoolers at risk. *Topics in Early Childhood Special Education, 27*, 232–249.

Volmink, J., Siegried, N., Robertson, K., & Gulmezoglu, A. M. (2004). Research synthesis and dissemination as a bridge to knowledge management: The Cochrane Collaboration. *Bulletin of the World Health Organization, 82*(10). Retrieved from http://www.ncbi.nlm.nih.gov/pmc/articles/PMC2623032/pdf/15643800.pdf

Walker, D., Bigelow, K., & Harjusola-Webb, S. (2008). Increasing communication and language-learning opportunities for infants and toddlers. *Young Exceptional Children Monograph Series #10*, 105–121.

Warren, S. F., Fey, M. E., Finestack, L. H., Brady, N. C., Bredin-Oja, S. L., & Fleming, K. K. (2008). A randomized trial of longitudinal effects of low-intensity responsivity education/prelinguistic milieu teaching. *Journal of Speech, Language, and Hearing Research, 51*(2), 451–470.

Warren, S. F., & Walker, D. (2005). Fostering early communication and language development. In D. M. Teti (Ed.), *Handbook of research methods in developmental science* (pp. 249–270). Malden, MA: Blackwell.

Wasik, B. H., Ramey, C. T., Bryant, D. M., & Sparling, J. J. (1991). A longitudinal study of two early intervention strategies: Project CARE. *Child Development, 61*, 1682–1696.

Wesley, P. W., Buysse, V., & Keyes, L. (2000). Comfort zone revisited: Child characteristics and professional comfort with consultation. *Journal of Early Intervention, 23*, 106–115.

What Works Clearinghouse (WWC). (2010, April). *WWC intervention report: Dialogic reading*. U.S. Department of Education, Institute for Educational Sciences (IES).

White, J. L., & Kratochwill, T. R. (2005). Practice guidelines in school psychology: Issues and directions for evidence-based interventions in practice and training. *Journal of School Psychology, 43,* 99–115.

Whitehurst, G. J., Arnold, D. S., Epstein, J. N., & Angell, A. L. (1994). A picture book reading intervention in day care and home for children from low-income families. *Developmental Psychology, 30*(5), 679–689.

Wolery, M. (2005). DEC recommended practices: Child-focused practices. In S. Sandall, M. L. Hemmeter, B. J. Smith, & M. E. McLean (Eds.), *DEC recommended practices: A comprehensive guide for practical application in early intervention/early childhood special education* (pp. 71–106). Longmont, CO: Sopris West.

Wolery, M., & Bailey, D. B. (2002). Early childhood special education research. *Journal of Early Intervention, 25,* 88–99.

Yoder, P., & Stone, W. (2006). A randomized comparison of the effect of two prelinguistic communication interventions on the acquisition of spoken communication in preschoolers with ASD. *Journal of Speech, Language, and Hearing Research, 49,* 698–711.

Yoder, P. J., & Warren, S. F. (2001). Relative treatment effects of two prelinguistic communication interventions on language development in toddlers with developmental delay vary by maternal characteristics. *Journal of Speech, Language, and Hearing Research, 44,* 224–237.

Chapter 7

Professional Development in Early Childhood Intervention: Emerging Issues and Promising Approaches

Patricia A. Snyder, Maria K. Denney, Cathleen Pasia, Salih Rakap, and Crystal Crowe

The critical role of professional development (PD) for ensuring high-quality early care and education that supports the development and learning of all young children is well documented (Bogard & Takanishi, 2005; Winton, McCollum, & Catlett, 2008; Zaslow & Martinez-Beck, 2006). The need to provide systematic, sustained, and evidence-informed professional development has become more urgent as demands for qualified early childhood personnel have increased and the body of knowledge has grown about dimensions of early childhood program quality and effective early childhood practices. In addition, contemporary early childhood quality improvement and accountability systems place significant emphasis on the role of professional development for equipping practitioners with knowledge, skills, and dispositions associated with improved learning outcomes for children and families (Harbin, Rous, & McLean, 2005; Schultz & Kagan, 2007).

Access to high-quality and effective early childhood professional development has not kept pace with the growing recognition of its significance. The Committee on Early Childhood Pedagogy reported that PD for early childhood practitioners is limited, inconsistent, and fragmented (Bowman, Donovan, & Burns, 2000). Investigators associated with the National Professional Development Center on Inclusion (2008) noted early childhood professional development efforts at local, state, and national levels often are uncoordinated, and until recently, no agreed-upon definition of early childhood professional development existed. During a recent federally sponsored listening-and-learning tour

(http://www.ed.gov/blog/2010/04/experts-discuss-the-early-learning
-workforce) designed to gather information about key issues in early
learning, experts identified three key priorities for improving early
childhood workforce quality: (1) better preparation, (2) support
for ongoing professional development, and (3) higher rewards and
compensation.

Specific to the preparation of early childhood practitioners who
support young children with disabilities and their families, the Center
to Inform Personnel Preparation Policy and Practice in Early Intervention and Preschool Education (2007a, 2007b) found that only 39 percent
of Part C early intervention programs and 58 percent of Section 619
preschool programs across 50 states, the District of Columbia, and
two territories had a systemic, sustainable approach to professional
development. Further, only 23 percent of Part C and 42 percent of
Section 619 programs had a comprehensive technical assistance system in place to support ongoing professional development (Bruder,
Mogro-Wilson, Stayton, & Dietrich, 2009).

Early childhood personnel often report they lack confidence and
competence to serve young children with disabilities in inclusive settings (Buysse, Wesley, Keys, & Bailey, 1996; Center to Inform Policy
and Practice in Early Intervention and Preschool, 2007c, 2007d). In
addition, early childhood teachers report they are not adequately prepared in their preservice programs for serving children with disabilities (Chang, Early, & Winton, 2005).

In the 25 years since the passage of P.L. 99-457 in 1986, services and
supports for infants, toddlers, and preschool children with disabilities
and their families have grown exponentially. All 50 states, the District
of Columbia, and two territories provide services and supports to eligible young children with disabilities and their families beginning at
birth. With this growth has come the development and definition of
early childhood intervention (birth to age 5) as a specialized area of
study and focused professional development. Although typically
referred to as early intervention/early childhood special education,
in this chapter, we use the term *early childhood intervention* broadly to
include supports and services provided to young children with or at
risk for disabilities and their families from birth to age 5.

The ages and unique needs of young children and their families, the
manner and settings in which young children learn, and a commitment
to inclusive, family-centered, and evidence-informed practices have
shaped the early childhood intervention field and its recommended
practices, including its recommended professional development

practices (Bruder et al., 2009; Crow & Snyder, 1998; Sandall, Hemmeter, Smith, & McLean, 2005; Sexton et al., 1996; Stayton, Miller, & Dinnebeil, 2002). Against this backdrop, the growing emphases on universally designed early childhood curricula, tiered prevention and intervention curricular frameworks, universal early learning standards, and early childhood accountability systems highlight the need to situate emerging issues and promising approaches to early childhood intervention professional development within broader early childhood professional development frameworks (Snyder, McLaughlin, & Denney, in press).

The purpose of this chapter is to consider emerging issues and promising approaches in early childhood intervention professional development. We begin the chapter by describing issues influencing the design, delivery, and evaluation of early childhood intervention professional development. Next, we review contemporary definitions for professional development that have emerged in early childhood. We analyze features of professional development hypothesized to be effective for supporting practitioners' application of knowledge, skills, and dispositions in practice contexts, which in turn affect child learning and development. We summarize findings from a systematic review of the empirical literature designed to characterize key features of early childhood professional development. We consider promising approaches to professional development in early childhood. These approaches focus explicitly on practitioners' implementation of evidence-based practices, and they are designed to lead to young children experiencing high-quality learning environments and instruction to support or accelerate their development and learning. We discuss frameworks and theories of action useful for guiding decisions about aligning professional development content, instructional approaches, and desired professional development outcomes. Finally, we consider key issues related to the future of early childhood intervention professional development.

EMERGING ISSUES RELATED TO EARLY CHILDHOOD INTERVENTION PROFESSIONAL DEVELOPMENT

At least six issues are important to consider with respect to ensuring better preparation of and ongoing professional development support for early childhood intervention practitioners: (1) cross-sector early childhood professional development, (2) early childhood standards and accountability systems, (3) diversity of children and families involved in early care and education programs, (4) tiered prevention and intervention curricular frameworks, (5) workforce issues, and (6) professional development leadership in early childhood intervention. Although in-depth consideration of each issue is beyond the scope of this chapter, it is important to review these issues briefly because they impact the design, delivery, and evaluation of promising professional development approaches in early childhood intervention.

Cross-Sector Early Childhood Professional Development

Early childhood programs and services are often fragmented or loosely coupled across various sectors, including Early Head Start and Head Start, state-funded prekindergarten (pre-K), early care and education, maternal and child health, mental health, and Part C and Section 619 of the Individuals with Disabilities Education Act. As Bagnato (2006) noted, "no [universal] field of early childhood exists, let alone a system" (p. 616). As states and communities work to align and integrate services and supports for young children and families across various early childhood sectors, including those sectors that focus on young children with or at risk for disabilities, the design, delivery, and evaluation of cross-sector early childhood professional development will become increasingly important (Snyder, Crowe, & Woods, 2010; Winton & McCollum, 2008). Cross-sector initiatives consider what knowledge, skills, and dispositions practitioners must have to support high-quality inclusive experiences for young children with or at risk for disabilities and their families (Buysse & Hollingsworth, 2009). As these authors noted, "Combined with what we already know about program quality for young children in general, the dimensions of inclusive program quality along with specific intervention practices are needed to improve existing program standards and guide professional development on early childhood inclusion" (p. 120). Coordination and integration will be needed to ensure that cross-sector early childhood professional development systems support the initial preparation and ongoing development of a cadre of practitioners who have the knowledge, skills, and dispositions to support the development and learning of increasingly diverse young children, including children with or at risk for disabilities.

Early Childhood Standards and Accountability Systems

Early childhood standards and accountability systems have, by necessity, included attention to the knowledge, skills, and dispositions practitioners must have to design high-quality learning environments;

implement planned, intentional, and differentiated instruction; and monitor children's progress toward meeting standards and achieving desired outcomes. Many states have implemented career ladders or pathways that specify competencies early childhood practitioners should demonstrate as they obtain initial and more advanced certifications, degrees, credentials, or licensure to "qualify" them to assume particular roles within and across early childhood sectors (e.g., lead teacher in an early care and education program, Part C early intervention provider, or pre-K teacher in an inclusive public school classroom). These credentialing systems and career pathways often focus on early childhood and early childhood special education and do not include other disciplines involved in providing supports and services to young children and their families, particularly those personnel who support young children with or at risk for disabilities and their families in inclusive early learning settings (e.g., speech and language therapists, occupational therapists, physical therapists, school psychologists). Given the range of preparation levels and disciplines included under the broad heading of early childhood intervention practitioner, a critical need exists to identify what knowledge, skills, and dispositions are needed by which early childhood intervention practitioners and under what circumstances to design a "second-generation" professional development system (cf. Guralnick, 1997).

Diversity of Children and Families Involved in Cross-Sector Early Care and Education Programs

The diversity of children and families involved in cross-sector early care and education programs is well documented (National Association for the Education of Young Children, 2009). According to the Federal Interagency Forum on Child and Family Statistics (http://www.childstats.gov), racial and ethnic diversity in the United States continues to increase. In 2008, 56 percent of children in the United States were White, non-Hispanic; 22 percent were Hispanic; 15 percent were Black; 4 percent were Asian; and 5 percent were other races. The percentage of children who are Hispanic has increased faster than any other group, from 9 percent in 1980 to 22 percent in 2008. Although racial and ethnic data are important, they alone do not reflect fully the diversity of children and their families in the United States. Beyond race and ethnicity, children are diverse with respect to culture, language, ability, family structure and membership, and socioeconomic status. This diversity necessitates attention to designing early childhood professional development to ensure that practitioners, regardless of their preparation and backgrounds, are culturally responsive and competent. Lynch and Hanson (1998) defined cross-cultural competence as "the ability to think, feel, and act in ways that acknowledge, respect, and build upon ethnic, [socio]cultural, and linguistic diversity" (p. 49). Identifying professional development approaches effective for preparing and supporting practitioners to be cross-culturally competent has become increasingly important. In addition, professional development in early childhood intervention must address effective instructional practices for children from diverse backgrounds and abilities, including children whose home language is not English or who primarily speak a language other than English in the home (Buysse, Castro, & Peisner-Feinberg, 2010; Espinosa, 2010).

Tiered Prevention and Intervention Curricular Frameworks

The growing emphasis on tiered early prevention and intervention curricular frameworks and associated practices, which are designed to support and accelerate the growth and learning of all young children in inclusive early care and education settings, necessitates a shift in how professional development is designed, delivered, and evaluated. Those involved in early childhood intervention professional development recognize that programs and practices for young children with or at risk for disabilities will increasingly be situated within, not apart from, the broader array of programs and practices for young children and their families (Snyder et al., in press; VanDerHeyden & Snyder, 2006). This means contemporary approaches to early childhood intervention professional development must include attention to dimensions of environmental and instructional quality that are important for all children, for some children, and for individual children. Early childhood intervention practitioners must be able to use data to make informed decisions about the type, level, and intensity of supports and early learning experiences provided to young children based on their abilities, needs, and circumstances rather than categorical labels or eligibility criteria. Early childhood professional development approaches that support practitioners to implement evidence-based practices with fidelity and to use data to make decisions about support or intervention intensity will become increasingly important as tiered frameworks are implemented in early childhood settings (Snyder, Hemmeter, & Fox, 2010).

Workforce Issues

Professional development is one dimension of larger workforce issues in early childhood and early childhood intervention (Weiss, 2005–2006; Whitebook, 2010). Persistent and challenging workforce issues in early childhood and early childhood intervention exist, including wages and benefits, labor market dynamics, and recruitment and retention (Brandon & Martinez-Beck, 2006; Bruder et al., 2009). As workforce issues are addressed, they will be inextricably linked to professional development and early childhood quality improvement efforts. As Ramey and Ramey (2006) noted, it is not desirable to have a stable but unskilled workforce or to sacrifice the quality of early care and education provided to young children because of turnover issues. When discussing how to attract, train, and sustain a high-quality workforce they stated, "The key is that the highest priority has to be placed on the direct provision of high-quality [education] and care at all times, in all settings, for all children" (p. 362).

Early Childhood Professional Development Leadership

Winton and McCollum (2008) described a pressing need to consider the knowledge, skills, and dispositions needed by professional development leaders. These authors defined professional development leaders as including the faculty, consultants, trainers, mentors, and coaches who help mediate the transfer and application of early childhood professional development content. Winton and McCollum noted professional development leaders, at a minimum, should be expected to have advanced, cross-sector content knowledge in (1) early childhood and early childhood intervention, (2) evidence-based practices, (3) research-based teaching and intervention strategies for supporting young children's development and learning, (4) skills related to working with adult learners, and (5) the ability to implement effective professional development strategies with fidelity. One unique challenge to be addressed by the next generation of professional development leaders is how to align PD across the various systems focused on early care and education. As more is learned about how to design, deliver, and evaluate cross-sector early childhood professional development, professional development leaders in early childhood intervention will be needed who can contribute meaningfully to its practice and research base.

DEFINING PROFESSIONAL DEVELOPMENT
IN EARLY CHILDHOOD

According to several widely respected sources, until recently, no agreed-upon definition for early childhood professional development existed (Maxwell, Feild, & Clifford, 2006; National Professional Development Center on Inclusion, 2008). Based on their review of 27 research studies focused on early childhood professional development, Maxwell et al. (2006) constructed definitions for various types of professional development, given there were no consistent definitions offered in the extant literature. These authors identified education, training, and credential as three types of professional development. *Education* was defined as professional development activities that occur within a formal education system. This often has been referred to in the literature as preservice training. *Training* was defined as professional development activities that occur outside the formal education system, which has often been characterized as in-service training. Finally, Maxwell et al. identified *credential* as a third type of professional development that does not fall into the education or the training category. These authors noted organizations that grant credentials such as early childhood teaching certifications or professional licensures often are not the same as those that deliver education and training, yet they play a key role in professional development systems.

To advance efforts related to developing a shared definition for early childhood professional development, investigators associated with the National Professional Development Center on Inclusion used iterative processes, including a review of the research literature and field review and validation, to construct a definition for professional development (Buysse, Winton, & Rous, 2009). The definition developed and disseminated by the Center is as follows: "Professional development is facilitated teaching and learning experiences that are transactional and designed to support the acquisition of professional knowledge, skills, and dispositions as well as the application of this knowledge in practice" (p. 3). As part of the conceptual framework that accompanies the definition, three key components of professional development were specified. These components focus on the *who*, the *what*, and the *how* of professional development. In addition, the framework specifies important infrastructure and contextual supports for early childhood professional development: (1) resources, (2) policies, (3) organizational structures, (4) access and outreach, and

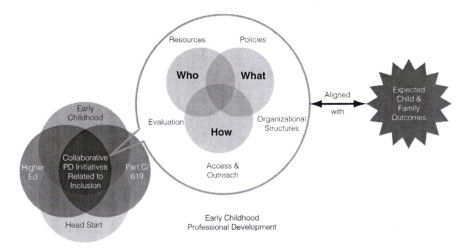

Figure 7.1   Conceptual framework for professional development in early childhood. Adapted from "The Big Picture: Building Cross-Sector Early Childhood Professional Development Systems" by C. Catlett & P. J. Winton, 2009, Smart Start Conference.

(5) evaluation. Figure 7.1 shows the NPDCI framework for early childhood professional development.

The *who* of professional development includes consideration of the characteristics and organizational contexts of learners and the characteristics and organizational contexts of those who design, deliver, and evaluate professional development. It also includes consideration of the characteristics and contexts of the diverse children and families with whom participants in professional development interact.

The *what* of professional development considers the content to be addressed or the knowledge, skills, or dispositions on which professional development is focused. To help determine what knowledge, skills, and dispositions are important for particular early childhood intervention practitioners and under what circumstances, guidance can be found by consulting professional competencies that specify core, specialized, and discipline-specific competencies (e.g., American Speech-Language-Hearing Association, 2008; Snyder, Crowe, & Woods, 2010; Thorp & McCollum, 1988); professional competencies or standards (e.g., Council for Exceptional Children, 2009; Division for Early Childhood, 2008); program quality standards or quality rating systems (Scott-Little, Cassidy, Lower, & Ellen, in press); child-focused early learning standards or guidelines (Scott-Little, 2010); and desired outcomes for children and families specified in early childhood accountability systems (Hebbeler, Barton, & Mallik, 2008).

The *how* of PD refers to the organization and facilitation of professional development experiences, including pedagogical or instructional strategies used to support teaching and learning. It includes consideration of promising instructional approaches that support the achievement of desired professional development outcomes (Snyder & Wolfe, 2008; Winton & McCollum, 2008), principles from adult learning (Knowles, 1984; Knowles, Holton, & Swanson, 1998) and the growing body of evidence related to how people learn (e.g., Bransford et al., 2000; Donovan, Bransford, & Pellegrino, 1999).

The definition of early childhood professional development developed and disseminated by the National Professional Development Center on Inclusion (NPDCI) emphasizes transactional and facilitated teaching and learning experiences and avoids dichotomizing two major categories of professional development that historically have developed somewhat independently (i.e., preservice and in-service training). One long-standing assumption has been that preservice training serves as an introduction to the world of practice, while in-service training develops, expands, or modifies the knowledge, skills, and dispositions of practitioners. Unfortunately, this dichotomy often is deleterious at the practice level in the development and maintenance of separate systems for preparing personnel to deliver early childhood intervention services (Sexton, Snyder, Lobman, Kimbrough, & Matthews, 1997). The emphasis on transactional and facilitated teaching and learning experiences in the NPDCI definition is useful for advancing broader conceptualizations of early childhood professional development and the types of activities that might be characterized as forms of professional development. The definition highlights the need not only to describe the types of professional development available in a comprehensive early childhood professional development system, but to consider systematically the who, what, and how of professional development and necessary infrastructure and contextual supports. Moreover, this definition can be used to support the development, implementation, and evaluation of "second-generation" early childhood professional development that considers which transactional and facilitated teaching and learning experiences focused on what knowledge, skills, and dispositions are needed by which early childhood intervention practitioners and under what circumstances. Of particular relevance to early childhood intervention is the identification of promising professional development features that support practitioners to implement evidence-based practices with fidelity in inclusive early learning settings and link practitioners' implementation of these practices to desired child and family outcomes.

FEATURES OF EFFECTIVE PROFESSIONAL DEVELOPMENT

Despite decades of literature documenting limitations associated with what has been referred to as the "train and hope," "spray and pray" or "one-shot" workshop approach to professional development, much of what occurs as professional development continues to be this approach. This professional development approach often involves a workshop session or two focused on raising awareness or gaining knowledge about a practice or set of practices; limited interactions among trainers and participants; little preparation or follow-up provided for participants; and a lack of consideration for learners' needs, experiences, and opportunities in relation to the professional development topic (Snyder & Wolfe, 2008). These features of professional development generally would be characterized as ineffective for supporting a theory of action or change related to desired relationships among high-quality professional development, practitioners' knowledge and skills related to evidence-based practices, the application of practitioners' knowledge and skills as reflected in intentional teaching and high-quality instruction, and child engagement and learning. Figure 7.2 shows a schematic that illustrates these hypothesized relationships.

In contrast to traditional approaches, contemporary perspectives about early childhood professional development reflect systematic attention to examining the relationships shown in Figure 7.2. This contemporary approach includes identifying and measuring features of professional development provided to practitioners and associating these features with improved fidelity of implementation of evidence-based practices and, in turn, positive outcomes for children and families.

A large body of anecdotal professional development literature, federal policy (e.g., No Child Left Behind Act of 2001; Good Start, Grow Smart Interagency Workgroup, 2005) and accumulating empirical evidence (Yoon, Duncan, Lee, Scarloss, & Shapley, 2007), including research related to how people learn (e.g., Bransford et al., 2000), has identified features of effective professional development. As Snyder and Wolfe (2008, p. 15) noted, effective professional development is

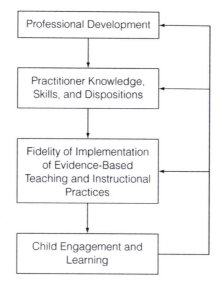

Figure 7.2 Theory of action or change illustrating desired relationships among high-quality professional development; practitioners' knowledge, skills, and dispositions related to evidence-based practices; the application of practitioners' knowledge and skills as reflected in intentional teaching and high-quality instruction; and child engagement and learning.

distinguished from ineffective professional development by its emphasis on coherency, research-based practices, and capacity building.

In K–12 education, consensus has emerged about features of effective professional development that are associated with student learning or achievement (Wayne, Yoon, Zhu, Cronen, & Garet, 2008). These features have also been identified as those most likely to be related to child learning and improved outcomes for young children and their families (Landry, Swank, Smith, Assel, & Gunnewig, 2006; Neuman & Cunningham, 2009; Pianta, Mashburn, Downer, Hamre, & Justice, 2008; Sheridan, Edwards, Marvin, & Knoche, 2009; Snyder & Wolfe, 2008; Winton & McCollum, 2008; Whitebook, 2010).

In the No Child Left Behind (NCLB) Act of 2001 (§ 9101 p. 1963), five features (criteria) of high-quality professional development are specified: (1) sustained, intensive, and content focused to have a positive and lasting impact on classroom instruction and teacher performance; (2) aligned with and directly related to state academic content standards, student achievement standards, and assessments; (3) improves and increases teachers' subject-matter knowledge; (4) advances teachers' understanding of effective instructional strategies based on scientifically based research; and (5) regularly evaluated for effects on teacher effectiveness and student achievement. One-day or short-term workshops or conferences are specifically identified as not meeting the definition for high-quality professional development under NCLB.

Beyond NCLB, several organizations or groups have specified standards or recommended practices for professional development, including the Division for Early Childhood of the Council for Exceptional Children (Miller & Stayton, 2005), the National Association for the Education of Young Children (NAEYC, under revision), the Council of Chief State School Officers (http://www.nectac.org/~pdfs/topics/ecpractices/gsgs.pdf), and the National Staff Development Council (http://www.nsdc.org/standards/index.cfm). Across these organizations and groups, several themes have emerged related to features of effective professional development linked to student achievement or desired child and family outcomes. These themes include (1) sustained over time, (2) grounded in practice (job embedded), (3) linked to curriculum and instructional goals, (4) collaborative, (5) interactive, and (6) the provision of support and feedback in practice settings.

In addition to the features of high-quality professional development specified in NCLB and by professional organizations or groups, features of effective professional development have been identified in empirical studies or systematic reviews of the professional development literature. Although these studies involved teachers working in K–12 education programs, the features of effective professional development identified in these studies likely are relevant for those who design, implement, and evaluate professional development in early childhood.

Kennedy's (1998) systematic review of the effects on student achievement of professional development programs focused on math and science demonstrated support for the conclusion that a coherent content focus was an important feature of the professional development. When examining relationships between professional development and student achievement, Kennedy developed a classification system that differentiated four types of studies included in her systemic review. Group 1 professional development studies focused on teaching behaviors that could be applied across all subjects (e.g., lesson planning or grouping methods). Group 2 professional development studies focused on teaching behaviors applied to a particular subject. Although the behaviors had a generic quality, they were applicable to a subject. Group 3 studies focused on general guidance related to curriculum and instruction, and the professional development content focus was justified on the basis of how students generally learn. Finally, Group 4 professional development studies focused on how students learn subject matter content and how to assess student learning. This type of professional development provided knowledge about how students learn particular subjects, but did not offer specific guidance on practices for teaching a subject. Kennedy found that professional development programs focused on teachers' instructional behaviors that did not have an explicit content focus (i.e., Group 1 studies) demonstrated smaller influences on student achievement than did programs focused on teachers' knowledge of the subject matter, the curriculum, or how students learn subject-matter content.

Building on findings from the systematic review provided by Kennedy, a series of survey and case-study evaluations were conducted to identify key features of effective professional development (Birman, Desimone, Porter, & Garet, 2000; Garet, Porter, Desimone, Birman, & Yoon, 2001). The Garet et al. (2001) study involved a nationally representative sample of 1,027 mathematics and science teachers who self-reported their experiences and behavior following participation in a Title II Elementary and Secondary Act professional development activity. The professional development activity on which the teacher reported was selected using a systematic, hierarchical sampling strategy (Garet et al., 2001). In addition to the survey, as part of the larger national evaluation of the Title II professional development program, 6 exploratory case studies and 10 in-depth case studies in five states were conducted (Birman et al., 2000). Through this work, six features of professional development associated with student achievement were identified as promising practices. Although these features were identified in studies involving mathematics and science teachers, they are relevant to efforts focused on identifying features of effective professional development in early childhood intervention.

Table 7.1 lists and defines the six features of effective professional development described by Garet et al. (2001). These features have been organized under two dimensions: structural and core or substantive. Of note, these two dimensions are similar to the structural and process dimensions identified as key features when examining the quality of early childhood learning environments (cf. LaParo, Sexton, & Snyder, 1998). Three features of effective professional development are organized under the structural dimension: (1) form, (2) duration, and

Table 7.1   Six Features of Effective Professional Development Organized by Two Major Dimensions

Dimension	Feature	Definition
Structural	Form	Type of professional development characterized as reform versus traditional
	Duration	Includes number of hours participants spend in a professional development activity and time span over which the activity takes place
	Collective Participation	Involvement of groups of practitioners from the same program, school, department, subject, or grade level
Core or Substantive	Content Focus	Professional development focuses on specific curriculum or content rather than focus on general teaching methods (e.g., lesson planning, grouping methods)
	Active Learning	Professional development instructional processes include opportunities for learners to be engaged in meaningful analyses of teaching and learning including discussion, planning, observations, analyses, and practice with feedback
	Coherence	Professional development incorporates experiences consistent with the learners' goals; builds on previous knowledge and skills; provides opportunities for learners to discuss their experiences with others; and aligns with standards, curricula, accountability, and assessments relevant to the learners' practice context(s)

Note: Adapted from "What makes professional development effective? Results from a national sample of teachers," by M. S. Garet, A. C. Porter, L. Desimone, B. F. Birman, and K. S. Yoon, 2008, *American Educational Research Journal, 38*, pp. 919–920. Copyright 2008 by the American Educational Research Association.

(3) collective participation. Form refers to the type of professional development provided and whether it is traditional (e.g., short-term workshop or conference) or reform (e.g., communities of practice, mentoring, or coaching). Duration relates to dosage of professional development and includes the number of hours that participants spend in a professional development activity and the time span over which the activity takes place. Collective participation refers to the involvement of groups of practitioners from the same program, school, department, subject, or grade level in professional development as contrasted with the participation of practitioners with no logical or cohesive connection with one another.

Substantive or "core" features specified by Garet et al. included (1) content focus, (2) active learning, and (3) coherence. Content focus is consistent with Kennedy's (1998) findings and emphasize that professional development should have an explicit content focus versus a focus on general teaching methods such as lesson planning or instructional grouping methods (Birman et al., 2000). Content focus is related to the "what" of professional development reflected the NPDCI definition (National Professional Development Center on Inclusion, 2008). Active learning refers to professional development processes that include opportunities for learners to be engaged in meaningful analyses of teaching and learning, including discussion, planning, observations, analysis, and practice with feedback. Active learning strategies are based on accumulating evidence related to how learners acquire, master, and use knowledge and skills (Bransford et al., 2000; Donovan et al., 1999). Active learning is reflected in the "how" of professional development by NPDCI. Finally, coherence refers to the degree to which the professional development incorporates experiences that are consistent with the learners' goals, builds on previous knowledge and skills, provides opportunities for learners to discuss their experiences with others, and aligns with standards, curricula, accountability, and assessments relevant to the learners' practice context(s).

Characterizing effective professional development as including the two dimensions and six features described by Garet et al. (2001), Yoon and colleagues (2007) conducted a systematic review of the empirical literature to evaluate the strength of the evidence related to relationships between teacher professional development and student achievement. Assuming the effects of professional development on student achievement are mediated by teacher knowledge and practice in the classroom, the authors proposed a theory of action or change similar to the one shown in Figure 7.2. They hypothesized that professional development affects student achievement through three interrelated processes: (1) professional development must be high quality as reflected in its theory of action, including planning, implementation, and evaluation; (2) teachers who participate in high-quality professional development must have the motivation, belief, and skills to apply professional development content in their teaching and instructional practices; and (3) teaching and instruction, affected by high-quality professional development, impacts student achievement.

Yoon et al. (2007) noted that to substantiate the empirical link between professional development and desired outcomes (e.g., student achievement, child engagement and learning), studies must present high-quality empirical evidence supporting the hypothesized relationships among professional development, teacher learning and practice, and desired student or child outcomes. After reviewing 1,343 studies conducted between 1986 and 2006 focused on the effects of in-service professional development on student achievement, these authors found only nine studies that met the evidence standards established by the What Works Clearinghouse (http://ies.ed.gov/ncee/wwc). Five of the studies met the "without reservations" evidence standards; four met the "with reservations" standards. Six studies were published in peer-reviewed journals, and three were unpublished doctoral dissertations. Of the nine studies, five were randomized controlled-group experimental trials, and four were quasi-experimental studies. The average standardized mean difference effect size across the nine studies was 0.54 (range –0.53 to 2.39) and the improvement index (i.e., difference between the percentile rank of the intervention group mean and the 50th percentile representing the control group mean in the control group distribution) was 21.

With respect to the "who" of professional development, all nine studies involved elementary school teachers (K–5) and their students. Those providing the professional development were the primary authors of the nine studies or their affiliated researchers, and no train-the-trainer approaches were used. The content focus ("what" of professional development) in four of the studies focused on reading and language arts, two studies focused on mathematics, two other studies focused on mathematics and reading/language arts, one study focused on science, and one study involved content in mathematics, science, and reading/language arts. With respect to the "how" of the professional development, Yoon et al. found the studies "varied much more in content and substance than in form" (p. 12). They noted it was not possible to discern any systematic pattern between how professional development was provided and its subsequent effects on student achievement because of the lack of variability in form and the significant variability in the duration and intensity of the professional development across a small number of studies.

Nevertheless, with respect to features of effective professional development, each of the nine studies involved a coherent set of workshops or summer institutes. Eight studies included some type of follow-up to support application of PD content. Follow-up activities ranged from one follow-up meeting after a four-week workshop in one study, to 13 follow-up meetings after a weeklong summer workshop. The number of contact hours ranged from 5 to 100 and the duration of the PD ranged from 4 weeks to 10 months. Yoon et al. found that studies that had greater than 14 hours of PD showed a positive and statistically significant effect on student achievement, while the three studies that had fewer hours of professional development (i.e., 5 to 14 hours) demonstrated no statistically significant effects on student achievement.

Anecdotal reports, statements from professional organizations, descriptions of recommended practices, and a growing body of empirical evidence have identified promising features of effective professional development. These features are particularly relevant for contemporary approaches to professional development in early childhood intervention that emphasize fidelity of implementation of evidence-based teaching and instructional practices to support young children's learning and development. Although consensus has been reached about key features of effective professional development, sufficient specificity is not available to confidently guide professional development practices (Yoon et al., 2007).

Specific to early childhood professional development, Sheridan et al. (2009) and Zaslow (2009) have emphasized the need to describe with greater specificity the underlying processes associated with effective professional development. Sheridan et al. noted the science of early childhood professional development necessitates specifying theories of action and examining evidence not only about the form of professional development (i.e., methods, structures, delivery approaches) but about processes or mechanisms associated with desired proximal (practitioner) and distal (child and family) outcomes. Zaslow described these mechanisms as "active ingredients" and asserted that to examine fully these ingredients, particularly in relation to desired outcomes, changes will be required in how the field conceptualizes and shares evaluations of early childhood professional development.

She noted that most reports of early childhood professional development focus primarily on structural features, including type or form, content focus, and dosage provided, but specify limited information about the nature of professional development activities, particularly sufficient and replicable descriptions of the mechanisms or active ingredients hypothesized to be associated with proximal or distal outcomes. A systematic review of the literature conducted by Snyder, Artman, Hemmeter, Kinder, and Pasia (2010) supported Zaslow's assertions about features of early childhood professional development that have been reported most often in the empirical literature. Findings from this review are discussed briefly in the next section.

FEATURES OF EARLY CHILDHOOD PROFESSIONAL DEVELOPMENT REPORTED IN THE EMPIRICAL LITERATURE

Snyder et al. (2010) conducted a systematic review of the empirical early childhood professional development literature to characterize key features using the NPDCI framework. These authors identified 235 empirical studies that involved a type of professional development specified on an investigator-developed coding form (see Table 7.2). In addition, the included studies had to involve early childhood practitioners or practitioners in training and to report empirical evidence about outcomes associated with professional development for either the early childhood practitioner or the children with whom the practitioner worked. As part of the review, the authors summarized the type of professional development provided to early childhood practitioners, the content focus of the professional development (the "what"), which early childhood practitioners participated in professional development (the "who"), and under what circumstances. With respect to the "how" of professional development, Snyder et al. were particularly interested in characterizing if follow-up teaching and learning strategies were used, particularly in-situ experiential strategies described as holding the most promise for supporting application of skills in practice contexts (i.e., coaching or consultation with performance feedback, mentoring, peer support groups, communities of practice or shared inquiry groups; Sheridan et al., 2009; Snyder & Wolfe, 2008). For studies that included the provision of feedback to support skill application, the authors summarized data-related structural and process mechanisms, including the feedback agent; the format for delivery of feedback; and the type, intensity, and duration of feedback provided. In addition, they

Table 7.2   Forms and Definitions of Professional Development Reflected in the Early Childhood Empirical Literature

Form of Professional Development	Definition
Staff Development	Training provided *on-site* to an *individual or group who works together* at a targeted program, facility, or school system. This takes the form of an on-site workshop or series of on-site workshops. This training may also include a needs assessment or follow-up component.
In-Service Training	Training provided to an individual or group in a structured setting *outside their regular work setting*. This takes the form of an off-site workshop or series of off-site workshops. This training may also include a needs assessment component or follow-up component.
Preservice Training	Training provided to teachers, interns, student teachers, practicum students, or paraprofessionals who are enrolled in coursework for academic credit in a degree program located in a structured setting. This includes preservice internship, practicum, or student teaching where participants receive academic credit.
In-situ Consultation and Coaching	Professional development takes place in practice contexts (i.e., in the classroom, in the home for early intervention providers). Learners receive "on-the-job" experiences, coaching, or feedback but no formal instruction or training occurs outside the practice context. Participants may receive continuing education credit for the experiences, but they are not enrolled in formal preservice academic coursework.
Induction/Mentoring	Professional development conducted on-site for novice professionals or paraprofessionals who have less than three years experience. Professional development is conducted by a teacher or another professional working in the same program.
Web Training	Course or workshop accessed via the Internet. The course or workshop may include interaction (electronic, by phone, or face-to-face via videoconferencing) between trainer and trainee.
Materials Only	Manuals, CDs, or other materials (textbooks, self-guided modules) provided to participant. No organized, formal training or follow-up is provided.
Shared Inquiry	Emphasis is on collaborative inquiry and reflection about learning. Learners work in groups to identify

(Continued)

Table 7.2   (Continued)

Form of Professional Development	Definition
	professional development needs and develop learning plans to meet these needs. May include identification or assessment of learning outcomes. Typically, there is limited involvement by "experts" or individuals who are not regular group members.
Other	Organized teaching or learning experiences not reflected in the categories listed above.

examined whether fidelity of implementation associated with the provision of feedback was evaluated.

With respect to the type of professional development provided, more than half of the 235 studies were characterized as providing staff development or inservice training (see Table 7.2 for definitions). Participants in the studies were identified as early childhood educators (78 studies), child care providers (74 studies), Head Start practitioners (67 studies), early childhood special educators (26 studies), early intervention providers (19 studies), kindergarten teachers (18 studies), family care providers (13 studies), and Early Head Start practitioners (7 studies). None of the studies reported including family members as participants in the professional development. Most often, professional development content focused on social-emotional development and challenging behaviors (62 studies) and pre-academic skills (49 studies).

Of the 235 studies that met the inclusion criteria, 185 reported using follow-up strategies as a component of the professional development intervention. In 134 of these studies, in-situ experiential strategies described as holding the most promise for supporting application of skills in practice contexts were implemented. In 108 studies, coaching with feedback was provided. Mentoring was used in 12 studies, peer support groups in 4 studies, and shared inquiry/communities of practice in 2 studies. The majority of individuals involved in organizing the experiential professional development activities were research staff or consultants, but their qualifications were described in only half of the reviewed studies. The length of time the experiential learning activities were implemented was not described in 33 percent of the studies. The most frequently occurring time category of was 7–12 months (22% of studies) and often was linked to a school year. Only 21 percent of the studies reported the experiential learning strategies extended over more than one school year. Experiential activities were most often implemented weekly (31% of studies) or monthly (16% of studies), although 37 percent of the studies did not describe the frequency of contact. The duration of each experiential activity was not specified in 56 percent of the studies, and the most frequently reported duration was 30 minutes or longer (27% of studies).

Verbal and written performance feedback was provided to participants in 56 and 26 of the 134 studies, respectively. Problem-solving discussion and goal setting was reported in 36 studies, and goal setting occurred in 25 studies. Most feedback was provided immediately following the experiential learning activity (48% of the studies), although delayed face-to-face feedback was provided in 24 percent of the studies. Feedback via the Web was provided in 7 percent of the 134 studies.

With respect to fidelity of implementation of the experiential strategy, 113 (84%) of the studies did not present fidelity data. The protocol used to implement the experiential strategy was also not described in 81 percent of the studies. Twelve studies indicated they followed a coaching manual. Overall, very limited information was provided about the mechanisms or active ingredients associated with the experiential learning activities.

PROMISING APPROACHES TO EARLY CHILDHOOD INTERVENTION PROFESSIONAL DEVELOPMENT

The review of the professional development literature by Snyder, Artman, et al. (2010) highlighted that early childhood professional development comes in different forms. It can be characterized by a variety of purposes, participants, contexts, methods, and desired outcomes. For example, professional development in early childhood intervention might be an awareness-level workshop about a new Part C provision under the Individuals with Disabilities Education Act. Alternatively, it might be a comprehensive program-wide initiative to support young children's social-emotional development and prevent challenging behaviors (e.g., Hemmeter, Fox, Jack, Broyles, & Doubet, 2007), a semester-long course on early childhood assessment, or an coherent series of workshops followed by sustained coaching to support application of evidence-based practices in an inclusive early learning program (Snyder, Hemmeter, Sandall, & McLean, 2008). The who, the what, and the how of the professional development (National Professional

Development Center on Inclusion, 2008) are likely to vary across these forms, as are the desired outcomes.

Desired learner outcomes targeted in early childhood professional development might include (1) raising awareness, (2) acquiring or enhancing knowledge, (3) acquiring or enhancing skills, or (4) shaping or modifying dispositions. Sheridan et al. (2009) noted these outcomes might be associated with changes in teachers' interactions with children or families, the design of high-quality learning environments, the use of specific curricular or teaching strategies for particular groups of children or an individual child, or other specific behaviors or meaningful targets.

When considering promising approaches to professional development in early childhood intervention, it is important to map backward from desired outcomes (Guskey, 2002) and to align structural and process features with the desired outcomes. The widely cited work of Joyce and Showers (2002) highlights limitations associated with professional development that involves only presentation of theory without opportunities for modeling, skill practice, and coaching for implementation. As shown in Table 7.3, by extrapolating from their research on effective staff development in relation to practitioners' "executive implementation" in practice contexts and subsequent effects on student achievement, Joyce and Showers predicted the

Table 7.3 Professional Development Components and Attainment of Outcomes in Terms of Percent of Participants

Components of PD	Participants Attaining Professional Development Outcomes		
	Knowledge	Skill	Transfer (Executive Implementation)
Presentation of Theory and Content	10%	5%	0%
Plus Demonstration and Modeling	30%	20%	0%
Plus Practice with Feedback	60%	60%	5%
Plus Coaching for Implementation in Practice Context	95%	95%	95%

Note: Adapted from "Student achievement through staff development," by B. R. Joyce and B. Showers, 2002, p. 78. Copyright 2002 by the American Society for Curriculum and Development.

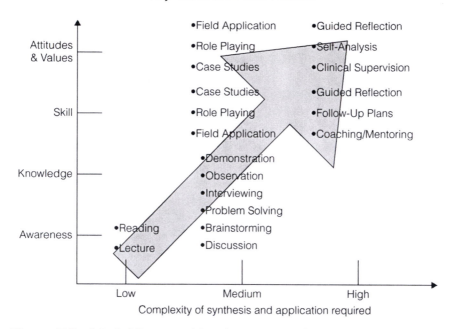

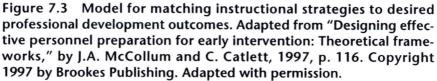

Complexity of synthesis and application required

Figure 7.3   Model for matching instructional strategies to desired professional development outcomes. Adapted from "Designing effective personnel preparation for early intervention: Theoretical frameworks," by J.A. McCollum and C. Catlett, 1997, p. 116. Copyright 1997 by Brookes Publishing. Adapted with permission.

percentages of participants likely to attain outcomes of knowledge, skill, or transfer (i.e., executive implementation) when various professional development components are implemented. These authors stated, "Note that the estimates are very rough, but they give rules of thumb for estimating the product of training" (p. 78).

McCollum and Catlett (1997) presented a framework that aligned various pedagogical or instructional strategies with desired professional development outcomes. As shown in Figure 7.3, this framework illustrates how instructional strategies (e.g., reading, case study, and self-reflection) should be considered with respect to both their complexity and the desired training outcome. For example, if the desired PD outcome is that practitioners will be aware of a new Part C regulation related to the natural-environments provision of IDEA, then a reading or self-guided instructional module on a Part C Web site might be an appropriate instructional strategy to achieve the desired awareness outcome. If, however, the desired outcome of professional development is focused on skill implementation in practice contexts, then more complex instructional strategies, including those identified by Joyce and Showers (2002) and the promising experiential learning strategies identified in the early childhood professional development literature, will be needed. These experiential strategies include coaching (Hanft, Rush, & Shelden, 2004), consultation (Buysse & Wesley, 2005), shared inquiry (Dana & Yendol-Hoppey, 2008), and communities of practice (Helm, 2007; Wesley & Buysse, 2006).

Despite growing consensus about features of effective professional development, results of the Yoon et al. (2007) systematic review and commentaries specific to early childhood PD by Sheridan et al. (2009) and Zaslow (2009) suggest the empirical evidence to date is limited with respect to professional development features (i.e., active ingredients) that make a difference in relation to desired proximal and distal outcomes (Wayne et al., 2008). Additional research is needed to guide the growing investments being made in professional development both in K–12 systems and in early childhood.

Wayne et al. (2008) suggested future professional development research be designed to address two main questions: (1) whether professional development programs that have demonstrated efficacy when implemented by study authors in controlled conditions remain effective when delivered by others under routine conditions, and (2) what specific features of professional development appear to matter most with respect to teaching and instructional practice and subsequent effects on student achievement. In addition, these authors noted a major challenge in that most professional development interventions involve at least two theories of action, which they characterized as a *theory of instruction* and a *theory of teacher change*. Wayne et al.'s two-theory analogy has utility for those who plan and implement professional development in early childhood intervention and for those who evaluate promising professional development approaches.

A *theory of instruction* represents the hypothesized links among the specific practitioner knowledge, skills, or dispositions emphasized in professional development, practitioners' implementation of teaching and instruction, and student achievement (Wayne et al., 2008). To illustrate a theory of instruction specific to early childhood intervention, we use an example from a project funded by the Institute of Education Sciences. This project is examining the impact of professional development on preschool teachers' use of embedded instruction practices (Snyder et al., 2008). The theory of instruction posited is that professionals focused on planning for, implementing, and evaluating embedded instruction (an evidence-based practice described by

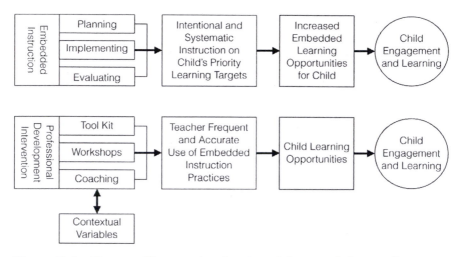

Figure 7.4   Theory of instruction (top) and theory of change (bottom) associated with professional development intervention focused on embedded instruction.

Wolery [2005]) will result in preschool teachers delivering more systematic and intentional instruction on priority learning targets to preschool children with disabilities in the context of activities, routines, and transitions in inclusive preschool settings. In turn, the investigators hypothesize that intentional instruction on priority learning targets will be associated with improvements in child learning and developmental outcomes. Figure 7.4 shows the theory of instruction for this professional development intervention.

Wayne et al. (2008) noted that a *theory of teacher or practitioner change* specifies the features of the professional development intervention hypothesized to promote change in teacher knowledge or practice, including the "mechanisms through which features of the professional development are expected to support teacher learning" (p. 472). This theory of change includes consideration of not only the structural features of the professional development identified by Garet et al. (i.e., form, duration, collective participation), but also the transactional teaching and learning experiences in which practitioners are involved and the intermediate or proximal practitioner outcomes the professional development experiences are expected to support.

In the Snyder et al. (2008) study, the theory of teacher change being examined is illustrated in Figure 7.4. The professional development emphasizes collective participation of 4–8 teachers working in preschool classrooms in a targeted program or school district. The investigators or personnel working with the investigators facilitate the professional development. The components of the intervention involve a series of coherent and content-focused workshops that are approximately 16 hours in duration. Active and experiential learning strategies are used in the workshops and include multiple-case and video exemplars of embedded instruction practices designed to guide learners' observations and analyses of practices. Workshop fidelity is evaluated systematically to ensure adherence to delivering the professional development as planned. Workbook and implementation practice guides are provided to each teacher along with a video camera that is used to record and analyze embedded instruction practices in the teacher's classroom during the series of workshops. With support from the workshop facilitator, teachers spend significant time during the workshop sessions engaged in case application activities related to planning for, implementing, and evaluating embedded instruction. Presently, the investigators are analyzing data related to which instructional strategies have been used in each workshop and how many minutes are spent using each strategy across sessions.

Coaching that includes performance feedback to support implementation of embedded instruction is an additional component of this professional development intervention. The coaching protocol includes a cyclical process that involves self-assessment related to embedded instruction implementation, goal setting and action planning, and monitoring and evaluation of implementation. Two variants of coaching are being examined: 15 weeks of in-situ coaching by an expert coach, or 15 weeks of self-coaching via a project-developed Web site. Both variants of coaching use the same cyclical coaching protocol, but coaching processes associated within each variant of coaching differ.

In the in-situ condition, coaching includes a 60-minute observation of the teacher in her classroom every other week for 15 weeks and an approximately 30-minute debriefing meeting that includes delivery of systematic performance feedback to the teacher about her frequent and accurate use of embedded instruction practices with targeted preschool children with disabilities. The feedback protocol used during debriefing includes the following six components: (1) open the feedback meeting, (2) provide supportive feedback, (3) provide corrective feedback, (4) provide targeted support, (5) discuss planned actions and needed resources or revise goals and action plan, and (6) close the feedback meeting. Debriefing, including feedback, is delivered face to face following each classroom observation and via e-mail, using the feedback protocol described above in each week that follows a scheduled observation. Coaches use a log for each in-situ and e-mail coaching session to report whether they implemented each component of the coaching and feedback protocols. They also report the strategies they used while conducting their observations and debriefings (e.g., modeling, reflective conversation, side-by-side gestural support) and the approximate time spent using each strategy. In addition to the coaches self-report of implementation, a second observer evaluates 33 percent of observation and debriefing sessions to evaluate adherence to the coaching and feedback protocols.

The intermediate practitioner outcomes of these professional development experiences are expected to support teachers' frequent and accurate use of embedded-instruction learning trials. One measure used to evaluate this proximal outcome is the Embedded Instruction Observation System (Snyder, Crowe, Hemmeter, Sandall, McLean, & Crow, 2009). Relationships between teachers' frequent and accurate implementation of embedded-instruction learning trials and child engagement and learning are also being evaluated.

We have used the Snyder et al. study as an exemplar to illustrate how a theory of instruction and a theory of teacher [practitioner] change described by Wayne et al. (2008) might be used to guide the design, implementation, and evaluation of promising PD approaches in early childhood intervention. Several other exemplars of PD studies, focused on promising approaches for supporting early childhood practitioners' implementation of evidence-based practices that can be linked to desired child learning outcomes, have appeared in the literature (e.g., Buysse et al., 2010; Hemmeter, Fox, & Snyder, 2008; Hemmeter, Snyder, Kinder, & Artman, in press; Hsieh, Hemmeter, McCollum, & Ostrosky, 2009; Landry et al., 2006; Neuman & Cunningham, 2009; Pianta et al., 2008). The professional development interventions implemented in these studies could be characterized with respect to the theories of instruction and teacher or practitioner change and the who, what, and how as reflected the NPDCI framework (NPDCI, 2008). Examining studies of early intervention professional development in this way would permit an analysis of the components of the professional development intervention and an evaluation of which practitioners received what professional development content, under which circumstances and in what dosage. In addition, these studies could be examined to identify whether associations were found between teachers' implementation of evidence-based practices and desired child outcomes. These studies and others will contribute importantly to the growing science of early childhood professional development.

THE FUTURE OF EARLY CHILDHOOD INTERVENTION PROFESSIONAL DEVELOPMENT

In 1997, Wolfe and Snyder noted that for too long, the train-and-hope mentality guided professional development in early childhood intervention. More than a decade later, although promising approaches to early childhood professional development are being increasingly implemented and systematically evaluated, we continue to witness a proliferation of one-shot workshops, Web-based training modules, and de-contextualized presentations by experts at national, state, and local conferences as though these are sufficient forms (and doses) of professional development. Although these approaches to professional development might achieve outcomes related to increasing awareness and knowledge, a growing body of evidence suggests they will not be associated with practitioners implementing evidence-based practices with fidelity or desired child and family outcomes.

Early childhood intervention professional development in the future must include content reflecting the latest information from the science of child development, particularly with respect to how to support the development and learning of young children with or at risk for disabilities. It must accommodate the diverse needs of children and families and reflect a second-generation orientation with respect to the adult learners who participate in and deliver the PD. Theories of action, including a theory of instruction and a theory of practitioner change, should be specified to guide PD planning, implementation, and evaluation. These theories of action should provide a depiction for all stakeholders and what, why, and how we do things (Bruder et al., 2009) and should help address important questions related to the growing science of early childhood professional development (Sheridan et al., 2009).

Early childhood intervention professional development in the future should incorporate instructional approaches that hold the most promise for achieving desired proximal outcomes (e.g., practitioners implementing evidence-based practices with fidelity) and distal outcomes (e.g., children who have positive social-emotional skills, take appropriate actions to meet their needs, and acquire and use knowledge and skills). These approaches will be based on what we know from the science of how people learn (Bransford et al., 2000), and from the growing body of empirical evidence related to active ingredients or features of effective PD (e.g., Joyce & Showers, 2002; Yoon et al., 2007).

Finally, early childhood intervention professional development of the future will be integrated within broader cross-sector initiatives occurring at local, state, and national levels. Duplicative and parallel early childhood professional development systems not only are inefficient, but are indefensible within current and projected fiscal and accountability climates (Bruder et al., 2009). If the intent of contemporary and future early childhood programs is to support positive outcomes for all young children and their families, then we must ensure that high-quality PD is provided to each practitioner who implements services and supports to young children with or at risk for disabilities and their families. This will require commitment and infrastructure supports from individuals representing many disciplines, agencies, and institutions at local, state, and national levels (Winton, McCollum, & Catlett, 2008). A cadre of leaders will be needed to advance the science and practice of early childhood intervention professional development. Fortunately, despite many challenges likely to be faced, promising approaches to early childhood intervention professional development are available to help guide these efforts.

REFERENCES

American Speech-Language-Hearing Association. (2008). *Core knowledge and skills in early intervention speech-language pathology practice*. Retrieved from http://www.asha.org/policy

Bagnato, S. J. (2006). Of helping and measuring for early childhood intervention: Reflections on issues and school psychology's role. *School Psychology Review, 35*, 615–620.

Birman, B. F., Desimone, L., Porter, A. C., & Garet, M. S. (2000). Designing professional development that works. *Educational Leadership, 57*, 28–33.

Bogard, K., & Takanishi, R. (2005). PK-3: An aligned and coordinated approach to education for children 3 to 8 years old. *Social Policy Report, 19*(3), 3–23. Retrieved from http://www.srcd.org/documents/publications/SPR/spr19-3.pdf

Bowman, B. T., Donovan, M. S., & Burns, M. S. (Eds.). (2000). *Eager to learn: Educating our preschoolers*. Report of the National Research Council, Committee on Early Childhood Pedagogy, Commission on Behavioral and Social Sciences and Education. Washington, DC: National Academy Press.

Brandon, R. N., & Martinez-Beck, I. (2006). Estimating the size and characteristics of the United States early care and education workforce. In M. Zaslow & I. Martinez-Beck (Eds.), *Critical issues in early childhood professional development* (pp. 49–76). Baltimore: Paul H. Brookes.

Bransford, J. D., Brown, A. L., Cocking, R. R., Donovan, M. S., Bransford, J. D., & Pelligrino, J. W. (Eds.). (2000). *How people learn: Brain, mind, experience, and school: Expanded edition*. Washington, DC: National Academy Press.

Bruder, M. B., Mogro-Wilson, C., Stayton, V. D., & Dietrich, S. (2009). The national status of in-service professional development systems for early intervention and early childhood special education practitioners. *Infants and Young Children, 22*(1), 13–20.

Buysse, V., Castro, D. C., & Peisner-Feinberg, E. (2010). Effects of a professional development program on classroom practices and outcomes for Latino dual language learners. *Early Childhood Research Quarterly, 25*, 194–206.

Buysse, V., & Hollingsworth, H. L. (2009). Program quality and early childhood inclusion: Recommendations for professional development. *Topics in Early Childhood Special Education, 29*, 119–128.

Buysse, V., & Wesley, P. W. (2005). *Consultation in early childhood settings*. Baltimore: Paul H. Brookes.

Buysse, V., Wesley, P. W., Keyes, L., & Bailey, D. B. (1996). Assessing the comfort zone of child care teachers in serving young children with disabilities. *Journal of Early Intervention, 20*, 189–204.

Buysse, V., Winton, P. J., & Rous, B. (2009). Reaching consensus on a definition of professional development for the early childhood field. *Topics in Early Childhood Special Education, 28*, 235–243.

Center to Inform Personnel Policy and Practice in Early Intervention and Preschool Education. (2007a, October). *Study VI data report: Training and technical assistance survey of state Part C coordinators*. Farmington: University of Connecticut, A. J. Pappanikou Center for Excellence in Developmental Disabilities, Education, Research, and Service, Author. Retrieved from http://www.uconnucedd.org/projects/per_prep/per_prep_resources.html

Center to Inform Personnel Policy and Practice in Early Intervention and Preschool Education. (2007b, October). *Study VI data report: Training and technical assistance survey of state Section 619 coordinators*. Farmington, CT: University of Connecticut, A. J. Pappanikou Center for Excellence in Developmental Disabilities, Education, Research, and Service, Author. Retrieved from http://www.uconnucedd.org/projects/per_prep/per_prep_resources.html

Center to Inform Personnel Policy and Practice in Early Intervention and Preschool Education. (2007c, October). *Study VII Part C data report: Competence and confidence of practitioners working with children with disabilities*. Farmington: University of Connecticut, A. J. Pappanikou Center for Excellence in Developmental Disabilities, Education, Research, and Service, Author. Retrieved from http://www.uconnucedd.org/projects/per_prep/per_prep_resources.html

Center to Inform Personnel Policy and Practice in Early Intervention and Preschool Education. (2007d, October). *Study VII Section 619 providers report: Competence and confidence of practitioners working with children with disabilities*. Farmington: University of Connecticut, A. J. Pappanikou Center for Excellence in Developmental Disabilities, Education, Research, and Service, Author.

Retrieved from http://www.uconnucedd.org/projects/per_prep/per_prep _resources.html

Chang, F., Early, D., & Winton, P. (2005). Early childhood teacher preparation in special education at 2- and 4-year institutions of higher education. *Journal of Early Intervention, 27*, 110–124.

Council for Exceptional Children. (2009). *What every special educator must know: Ethics, standards, and guidelines.* Arlington, VA: Author.

Crow, R. E., & Snyder, P. (1998). Organizational behavior management in early intervention: Status and implications for research and development. *Journal of Organizational Behavior Management, 18*(2–3), 131–156.

Dana, N. F., & Yendol-Hoppey, D. (2008). *The reflective educators guide to professional development: Coaching inquiry-oriented learning communities.* Thousand Oaks, CA: Corwin.

Division for Early Childhood. (2008). *Early childhood special education/early intervention (birth to age 8) professional standards with CEC common core.* Missoula, MT: Author. Available at http://www.dec-sped.org

Donovan, M. S., Bransford, J. D., & Pellegrino, J. W. (Eds.). (1999). *How people learn: Bridging research and practice.* Washington, DC: National Academy Press.

Espinosa, L. (2010). *Getting it right for young children from diverse backgrounds: Applying research to improve practice.* New York: Learning Solutions.

Garet, M. S., Porter, A. C., Desimone, L., Birman, B. F., & Yoon, K. S. (2001). What makes professional development effective? Results from a national sample of teachers. *American Education Research Journal, 38*, 915–945.

Good Start, Grow Smart Interagency Workgroup. (2005, December). *Good Start, Grow Smart: A guide to Good Start, Grow Smart and other federal early learning initiatives.* Retrieved from http://www.acf.hhs.gov/programs/ccb/initiatives/gsgs/fedpubs/GSGSBooklet.pdf

Guralnick, M. J. (1997). Second-generation research in the field of early intervention. In M. J. Guralnick (Ed.), *The effectiveness of early intervention* (pp. 3–22). Baltimore: Paul H. Brookes.

Guskey, T. R. (2002). Does it make a difference? Evaluating professional development. *Educational Leadership, 59*(3), 45–51.

Hanft, B., Rush, D., & Shelden, M. (2004). *Coaching families and colleagues in early childhood.* Baltimore: Paul H. Brookes.

Harbin, G., Rous, B., & McLean, M. E. (2005). Issues in designing state accountability systems. *Journal of Early Intervention, 27*, 137–164.

Hebbeler, K., Barton, L. R., & Mallik, S. (2008). Assessment and accountability for programs serving young children with disabilities. *Exceptionality, 16*(1), 48–63.

Helm, J. H. (2007). Energize your professional development by connecting with a purpose: Building communities of practice. *Young Children, 62*, 12–16.

Hemmeter, M. L., Fox, L., Jack, S., Broyles, L., & Doubet, S. (2007). A program-wide model of positive behavior support in early childhood settings. *Journal of Early Intervention, 28*, 337–355.

Hemmeter, M. L., Fox, L., & Snyder, P. (2008). *The Teaching Pyramid Observation Tool research edition.* Unpublished assessment.

Hemmeter, M. L., Snyder, P. A., Kinder, K., & Artman, K. (in press). Impact of performance feedback delivered via electronic mail on preschool teachers' use of descriptive praise. *Early Childhood Research Quarterly.*

Hsieh, W. Y., Hemmeter, M. L., McCollum, J. A., & Ostrosky, M. M. (2009). Using coaching to increase preschool teachers' use of emergent literacy teaching strategies. *Early Childhood Research Quarterly, 24,* 229–247.

Joyce, B., & Showers, B. (2002). *Student achievement through staff development* (3rd ed.). Alexandria, VA: Association for Supervision and Curriculum Development.

Kennedy, M. (1998). *Form and substance of inservice teacher education* (Research Monograph No. 13). Madison: National Institute for Science Education, University of Wisconsin.

Knowles, M. S. (Ed.). (1984). *Andragogy in action.* San Francisco: Jossey-Bass.

Knowles, M. S., Holton, E. F., & Swanson, R. A. (1998). *The adult learner: The definitive classic in adult education and human resource development* (5th ed.). Houston, TX: Gulf.

Landry, S. H., Swank, P. R., Smith, K. E., Assel, M. A., & Gunnewig, S. B. (2006). Enhancing early literacy skills for preschool children: Bringing a professional development model to scale. *Journal of Learning Disabilities, 39,* 306–324.

LaParo, K. M., Sexton, J. D., & Snyder, P. (1998). Program quality characteristics in segregated and integrated early childhood classrooms. *Early Childhood Research Quarterly, 13,* 151–167.

Lynch, E. W., & Hanson, M. J. (1998). *Developing cross-cultural competence: A guide for working with children and their families* (2nd ed.). Baltimore: Paul H. Brookes.

Maxwell, K. L., Feild, C. C., & Clifford, R. M. (2006). Defining and measuring professional development in early childhood research. In M. Zaslow & I. Martinez-Beck (Eds.), *Critical issues in early childhood professional development* (pp. 21–48). Baltimore: Paul H. Brookes.

McCollum, J. A., & Catlett, C. (1997). Designing effective personnel preparation for early intervention: Theoretical frameworks. In P. J. Winton, J. A. McCollum, & C. Catlett (Eds.), *Reforming personnel preparation in early intervention: Issues, models, and practical strategies.* Baltimore: Paul H. Brookes.

Miller, P. S., & Stayton, V. D. (2005). DEC recommended practices: Personnel preparation. In S. Sandall, M. L. Hemmeter, B. J. Smith, & M. E. McLean (Eds.), *DEC recommended practices: A comprehensive guide for practical application* (pp. 189–219). Longmont, CO: Sopris West.

National Association for the Education of Young Children. (2009). *Developmentally appropriate practice in early childhood programs serving children from birth through age 8* (Position statement). Retrieved from http://www.naeyc.org/files/naeyc/file/positions/PSDAP.pdf

National Professional Development Center on Inclusion. (2008). *What do we mean by professional development in the early childhood field?* Chapel Hill: University of North Carolina, FPG Child Development Institute. Retrieved from http://community.fpg.unc.edu/npdci

Neuman, S., & Cunningham, L. (2009). The impact of professional development and coaching on early language and literacy instructional practices. *American Educational Research Journal, 46,* 532–566.

No Child Left Behind Act of 2001, 20 U.S.C. § 9101 (2002).

Pianta, R. C., Mashburn, A. J., Downer, J. T., Hamre, B. K., & Justice, L. (2008). Effects of web-mediated professional development resources on teacher-child interactions in pre-kindergarten classrooms. *Early Childhood Research Quarterly, 23,* 431–451.

Ramey, S. L., & Ramey, C. T. (2006). Creating and sustaining a high-quality work-force in child care, early intervention, and school readiness programs. In M. Zaslow & I. Martinez-Beck (Eds.), *Critical issues in early childhood professional development* (pp. 355–368). Baltimore: Paul H. Brookes.

Sandall, S., Hemmeter, M. L., Smith, B. J., & McLean, M. E. (Eds.). (2005). *DEC recommended practices: A comprehensive guide for practical application in early intervention/early childhood special education.* Longmont, CO: Sopris West.

Schultz, T., & Kagan, S. L. (2007). *Taking stock: Assessing and improving early childhood learning and program quality.* New York: Foundation for Child Development.

Scott-Little, C. (2010, May). *Early learning standards: Variations across states and issues to consider.* Presentation at the Listening and Learning About Early Learning Tour, Chicago: Retrieved from http://www2.ed.gov/about/inits/ed/early learning/tour.html

Scott-Little, C., Cassidy, D. J., Lower, J., & Ellen, S. (in press). Early learning standards and program quality-improvement initiatives: A systematic approach to supporting children's learning and development. In P. W. Wesley & V. Buysse (Eds.), *Expanding program quality in early childhood: Raising the bar.* Baltimore: Paul H. Brookes.

Sexton, J. D., Snyder, P., Lobman, M. S., Kimbrough, P. M., & Matthews, K. (1997). A team-based model to improve early intervention programs: Linking preservice and inservice. In P. J. Winton, J. A. McCollum, & C. Catlett (Eds.), *Reforming personnel preparation in early intervention: Issues, models, and practical strategies* (pp. 495–526). Baltimore: Paul H. Brookes.

Sexton, J. D., Snyder, P., Wolfe, B., Lobman, M., Stricklin, S., & Akers, P. (1996). Early intervention inservice training strategies: Perceptions and suggestions from the field. *Exceptional Children, 62,* 485–495.

Sheridan, S. M., Edwards, C. P., Marvin, C. A., & Knoche, L. L. (2009). Professional development in early childhood programs: Process issues and research needs. *Early Education and Development, 20,* 377–401.

Snyder, P., Artman, K., Hemmeter, M. L., Kinder, K., & Pasia, C. (2010). *Characterizing key features of the early childhood professional development literature.* Manuscript in preparation.

Snyder, P., Crowe, C., Hemmeter, M. L., Sandall, S., McLean, M., & Crow, R. (2009). *EIOS: Embedded instruction for early learning observation system* [Manual and training videos]. Unpublished instrument. Gainesville: University of Florida.

Snyder, P., Crowe, C., & Woods, J. (2010). *Core inclusion competencies for early intervention and early childhood special education.* Manuscript in preparation.

Snyder, P., Hemmeter, M. L., & Fox, L. (2010, March). *Data based decision-making and the Pyramid Model: Are we doing what we should be doing and is it making a difference?* Presentation at the National Training Institute on Effective Practices: Supporting Young Children's Social Emotional Development, Clearwater Beach, FL. Available at http://www.challengingbehavior.org/do/training.htm

Snyder, P., Hemmeter, M. L., Sandall, S., & McLean, M. (2008). *Impact of professional development on preschool teachers' use of embedded instruction practices* [Abstract]. Washington, DC: Institute of Education Sciences. Retrieved from http://www.ed.gov/about/offices/list/ies/index.html

Snyder, P. A., McLaughlin, T., & Denney, M. K. (in press). Program focus in early childhood intervention. In J. M. Kauffman & D. P. Hallahan (Series Eds.) & M.

Conroy (Section Ed.), *Handbook of special education: Section XII Early identification and intervention in exceptionality.* New York: Routledge.

Snyder, P., & Wolfe, B. (2008). The big three process components of effective professional development: Needs assessment, evaluation, and follow-up. In P. J. Winton, J. A. McCollum, & C. Catlett (Eds.), *Practical approaches to early childhood professional development: Evidence, strategies, and resources* (pp. 13–51). Washington, DC: Zero to Three Press.

Stayton, V. D., Miller, P. S., & Dinnebeil, L. A. (Eds.). (2002). *DEC personnel preparation in early childhood special education: Implementing the DEC recommended practices.* Longmont, CO: Sopris West.

Thorp, E. K., & McCollum, J. A. (1988). Defining the infancy specialization in early childhood special education. In J. B. Jordan, J. J. Gallagher, P. L. Huntinger, & M. B. Karnes (Eds.), *Early childhood special education: Birth to three* (pp. 148–161). Reston, VA: Council for Exceptional Children.

VanDerHeyden, A. M., & Snyder, P. A. (2006). Integrating frameworks from early childhood intervention and school psychology to accelerate growth for all young children. *School Psychology Review, 35,* 519–534.

Wayne, A. J., Yoon, K. S., Zhu, P., Cronen, S., & Garet, M. S. (2008). Experimenting with teacher professional development: Motives and methods. *Educational Researcher, 37,* 469–479.

Weiss, H. (2005–2006). From the director's desk. *Evaluation Exchange, 11*(4), 1. Retrieved from http://www.hfrp.org/evaluation/the-evaluation-exchange/issue-archive

Wesley, P. W., & Buysse, V. (2006). Building the evidence based through communities of practice. In V. Buysse & P. W. Wesley (Eds.), *Evidence-based practice in the early childhood field* (pp. 161–194). Washington, DC: Zero to Three Press.

Whitebook, M. (2010, April). No single ingredient: 2020 vision for the early learning workforce. Paper presented at the Listening and Learning About Early Learning Tour, Denver, CO. Retrieved from http://www2.ed.gov/about/inits/ed/earlylearning/tour.html

Winton, P. J., & McCollum, J. A. (2008). Preparing and supporting high-quality early childhood practitioners: Issues and evidence. In P. J. Winton, J. A. McCollum, & C. Catlett (Eds.), *Practical approaches to early childhood professional development: Evidence, strategies, and resources* (pp. 1–12). Washington, DC: Zero to Three Press.

Winton, P. J., McCollum, J. A., & Catlett, C. (2008). *Practical approaches to early childhood professional development: Evidence, strategies, and resources.* Washington, DC: Zero to Three Press.

Wolery, M. (2005). Recommended practices: Child-focused practices. In S. Sandall, M. L. Hemmeter, B. J. Smith, & M. E. McLean (Eds.), *DEC recommended practices: A comprehensive guide for practical application* (pp. 71–106). Longmont, CO: Sopris West.

Wolfe, B., & Snyder, P. (1997). Follow-up strategies: Ensuring that instruction makes a difference. In P. Winton, J. McCollum, & C. Catlett (Eds.) *Reforming personnel preparation in early intervention: Issues, models, and practices* (pp. 173–190). Baltimore: Paul H. Brookes.

Yoon, K. S., Duncan, T., Lee, S. W., Scarloss, B., & Shapley, K. L. (2007). *Reviewing the evidence on how teacher professional development affects student achievement*

(Issues and Answers Report, REL-2007-No. 033). Washington, DC: U.S. Department of Education, Institute of Education Sciences, National Center for Educational Evaluation and Regional Assistance, Regional Educational Laboratory Southwest.

Zaslow, M. J. (2009). Strengthening the conceptualization of early childhood professional development initiatives and evaluations. *Early Education and Development, 20,* 527–536.

Zaslow, M. J., & Martinez-Beck, I. (2006). *Critical issues in early childhood professional development.* Baltimore: Paul H. Brookes.

Chapter 8

Crossing Systems in the Delivery of Services

Louise A. Kaczmarek

CROSSING THE COUNTY LINE: THE PRESBYLSKI FAMILY

The Presbylski family lives in Monroe County, very close to the border with Smithfield County. Michael Presbylski, age 4, has been attending the ABC Child Care Center, which is in Smithfield County, about a mile from the Presbylski home, since he was 6 months old. Teresa, Michael's sister, age 7, used to attend this child care center before she started kindergarten in her neighborhood school in Monroe County. John and Elizabeth Presbylski have been extremely pleased with the care their two children have received at the ABC Child Care Center. The location of the child care center has had the added benefit of convenience for the family. The youngest daughter, Carrie, age 2, who has Down syndrome, recently started to attend the ABC Child Care Center. Because of Carrie's special needs, John's mother had been taking care of Carrie at the Presbylski home; but at age 72, with Carrie's development into a very active toddler, she was unable to continue. Carrie has been receiving early intervention services at home, but with some issues that have arisen in child care, the Presbylskis would like the early intervention services to be delivered at ABC Child Care Center so that the early intervention staff can assist the child care staff in better meeting Carrie's needs. However, because the center is not in their county of residence, they will either have to forego receiving early intervention services at ABC Child Care Center, or they will have to find a child care center for Carrie in Monroe County.

WHO TO BELIEVE: THE GARZA FAMILY

Mr. and Mrs. Garza are confused. Their son Paco, who is 26 months of age, was diagnosed with autism at 20 months. Paco is receiving home-based services from two service agencies. Paco has two treatment plans—an Individualized Family Service Plan from the local early intervention agency, and a second treatment plan from behavioral health services. The developmental specialist from the Early Intervention Agency comes to the home once a week and wants the Garzas to be active in executing certain treatment strategies throughout the day with Paco. Soon Paco will also be receiving services from a speech-language pathologist also funded by the Early Intervention Agency, who will begin to teach Paco to use pictures as a means of communication. The Mental Health Center, on the other hand, provides 30 hours of intensive behavioral treatment, including teaching Paco to communicate using signs. There are two therapeutic staff personnel who administer a carefully designed regimen of programs to Paco in a special section of the family's basement six days a week for five hours each day. Although Mr. and Mrs. Garza get periodic updates from the supervisor every couple of weeks, the treatment at this stage requires that Paco's parents not be involved in any of the treatment. The Garzas just do not know what to do—one agency is telling them that their involvement is critical to the success of the treatment, and the other is implying that their involvement is contrary to successful treatment. One agency is advocating a communication method using picture cards, while the other is using signs. Mr. and Mrs. Garza, who have the utmost respect for both sets of professionals, just do not know how to resolve these contradictions. Although they are trying to implement the recommended early intervention strategies within their daily routines, they are finding that the best time for them to do it is after Paco's behavioral health sessions. However, Paco seems so exhausted from the intensive therapy that most of the time, he just ends up tantruming. They are trying to respect the wishes of each service agency, because they know how important the services are for Paco. Recently, they have begun to realize that they have not observed much progress in his behavior, particularly his communication in their daily lives.

    The cases of the Presbylski and Garza families demonstrate some of the difficulties that families may encounter in receiving services for their young children with disabilities. In the case of the Presbylski family, there is a conflict with the service regulations of the two early intervention providers. The services that would be most beneficial for the family are blocked by regulations that preclude service delivery across county lines. In the case of the Garza family, the child is receiving services from two different service systems—the educational system providing early intervention services, and the behavioral health system providing wraparound services. The child has two treatment plans that contradict each other, leaving the parents in a quandary about what is best for their child. In both cases, greater collaboration between the two service entities would better serve the needs of the families.

The purpose of this chapter is to identify the need for and the benefits of working across service boundaries in the delivery of services to young children with disabilities and their families and to examine how such collaborations are accomplished.

SYSTEMS OF SERVICE

Young children with disabilities and their families often have multiple needs and require multiple services from professionals, not only within the same service system, but also from other systems. Generally speaking, the more severe a child's disability or the more at risk a child's family, the more likely they are to need services from a variety of disciplines, agencies, and systems. Although services are provided by distinct entities, the services themselves may not necessarily be exclusive; consequently, services from one entity often impact those provided by another. For example, a child might be receiving speech and language services through their health care insurance plan as well as through the school district, the services for each being delivered by a different person following regulations for services in accordance with their specific service system. Neither system requires that one service provider talk to the other, so it could be, as was the case with the Garza family above, that the services can be directly contradictory. In other cases, services might simply not be sufficiently complementary to have the greatest impact on a child's progress. The parent is usually privy to the aims and methods of both. However, the inclusion of parents in making decisions about the goals of therapy, the methods to be used, and the role of parents in the therapy itself varies according to the service entity. Additionally, the dichotomous services require families to take on the role of service coordinator, since they are the common factor. We might broadly define these service systems as Health Care, Education, and Social Services, even though it is almost always true that a so-called "system" is in itself made up of multiple systems. In general, a system is a collection of parts that interact together and function as a whole (Ackoff & Rovin, 2003). Young children with disabilities are typically involved with many such systems.

A child may be receiving health care or aspects of health care through a private insurance plan, a public plan (e.g., Children's Health Insurance Program [CHIP], Medicaid), or a combination of both. Within health care, there are primary care providers and those providing specialized care. The type or the extent of services available will depend upon the nature of the insurance plan itself. There are also a number of other public programs that fall under the health sector. These include services under the Maternal and Child Health Block Grant (Title V), including programs for Children with Special Healthcare Needs and the program for Early and Periodic Screening and Diagnostic Treatment (EPSDT).

Within the educational realm, young children encounter other systems of services. They may be receiving early intervention services through Part C of IDEA if they are under 3 years of age and through Part B, Section 619 of IDEA if they are of preschool age. In some states these represent the same system and in others different systems. In addition to receiving early intervention services, a child might be attending a private or public child care center or preschool. For some, early intervention services might take place within the child care center itself, requiring two systems to interact with each other; for others, early intervention services and child care/preschool programs may be totally separate. Upon reaching school age, a child transfers to school-age services, which, depending upon the educational system delivering early intervention services, may or may not require a change in the educational entity. Children receiving early intervention services within a school district may simply need to transfer to school-aged services within the district, while those receiving early intervention from a private agency or other public unit may need to transfer into a completely new system.

Social services are probably the most complicated of all, because there are many types of services available; and even though they may fall under the same department in a state, such programs often operate in total isolation. Like Paco Garza, a child may be receiving mental or behavioral health services in addition to early intervention services, which in many states is considered an educational service. Additionally, children and their families may be receiving other types of social services such as Social Security income (SSI) for children with disabilities, family counseling, and home visiting services through Early Head Start or family support programs. Programs for other vulnerable populations also fall under social services and might include child protective services, Temporary Assistance for Needy Families (TANF), programs for the homeless and drug/alcohol abuse recovery, childcare subsidies, food (e.g., food stamps, WIC), and housing assistance programs.

LEGISLATIVE UNDERPINNINGS

Recognition of the needs and benefits of collaboration across programs, agencies, and systems spawned legislation to develop and formalize collaborative efforts within and across service entities.

Individuals with Disabilities Education Act (IDEA)

Interagency collaboration on behalf of young children with disabilities and their families was formalized in 1986 with the reauthorization of the Education of All Handicapped Children Act of 1986 (P.L. 99-457; California Department of Education, 2007). This act, which established the Program for Infants and Toddlers (Part H), required that agencies collaborate with one another in the delivery of services to this population and their families and that existing services for infants and toddlers not be supplanted by the establishment of new state programs. To assist in this effort, a National Interagency Coordinating Council was instituted and states that intended to develop an Infant-Toddler Program were required to create State Interagency Coordinating Councils (SICCs) consisting of 15 key representatives who had a stake in the delivery of services, including service providers, state-level administrators, and parents. The purpose of the SICCs, which are independent, multidisciplinary, and cross-systemic, is to advise and assist the lead public agency responsible for early intervention in the development, implementation, and evaluation of a well-coordinated service system (Harbin & Van Horn, 1990; Peterson, 1991).

The focus on interagency collaboration, especially in the Infant-Toddler Program (now referred to as Part C), has continued to be a strong focus in each reauthorization of this legislation. The most recent reauthorization in 2004, under the title of the Individuals with Disabilities Education Improvement Act (IDEIA; P.L. 108-446, 2004), contained a number of changes relating to interagency collaboration, further strengthening the requirements for collaboration with agencies serving specific populations such as homeless children and their families and children who are wards of the state. The reauthorization required the referral of children for evaluation who experience a substantiated case of trauma due to family violence. Additionally, the legislation called for early intervention screening, with referral for evaluation as appropriate, for children involved in substantiated cases of child abuse or neglect, those affected by illegal substance abuse, or those demonstrating withdrawal symptoms from prenatal drug exposure. Although the legislation abolished the National Interagency Coordinating Council, it required the appointment of several new members to State Interagency Coordinating Councils, namely a representative from the state Medicaid agency, the office of the Coordinator of Education of Homeless Children and Youth, the state child welfare agency, and the state agency responsible for children's mental health. Under the Part C program, states must also report their efforts to promote collaboration among Head Start programs, early education, and child care programs. More explicit requirements were specified for interagency agreements to ensure fiscal responsibility and for the continuation of services to children and families while resolving disputes about services (i.e., pendency).

Head Start Act

Head Start legislation, which has mandated the inclusion of children with disabilities since 1972, has also over the years strengthened its mandates for collaboration with other agencies and programs. The 1990 reauthorization of Head Start legislation established the first wave of Head Start Collaboration grants and established the State Head Start Collaboration Offices (Office of Head Start, 2007). The 1998 reauthorization identified eight priority areas for collaboration. The most recent Head Start Act, passed in 2007, requires enhanced collaboration and cooperation of Head Start agencies with a wide range of other entities that are devoted to benefiting low-income children from birth to school entry and their families. Through the legislation, collaboration grants are awarded to states for collaborative activities with other entities such as early care and education, health care, mental health care, welfare, child protective services, services relating to children with disabilities, English-language learners, homeless children, and family literacy programs. The legislation also urges the alignment of Head Start and state early learning standards. States receiving a collaboration grant must appoint a Director of Head Start Collaboration and convene a State Advisory Council on Early Childhood Education and Care consisting of representatives from a variety of service entities.

Keeping Children and Families Safe Act

In 2003, Congress passed the Keeping Children and Families Safe Act (P.L. 108-36), which reauthorized the Child Abuse Prevention and Treatment Act (P.L. 104-235; 1996) and several other acts (National Association of Social Workers, 2003). Like IDEIA, this act also requires states to refer infants and toddlers involved in a substantiated case of child abuse or neglect to early intervention for screening and, as appropriate, evaluation. It also strengthens interagency collaboration in services to children who are abused or neglected by allowing grant funding to be used for coordinating and obtaining services, including financial assistance and health and social services, for families with infants who have disabilities with serious life-threatening conditions. The act further encourages in its research, technical assistance, and demonstration projects interagency linkages to better ensure that children who have been abused or neglected have their physical health, mental health, and developmental needs assessed and treated.

Child and Adolescent Service System Program (CASSP)

After recognizing that children and adolescents with severe emotional disturbance were drastically under- and inadequately served by a fragmented and uncoordinated service system, the National Institute of Mental Health launched the Child and Adolescent Service System Program in 1984 (CASSP; Kysor, 1995). The program not only makes available needed services, but specifically encourages states and local communities to develop comprehensive systems of services that were child-centered, family-focused, community-based, multi-system, and least restrictive. This requires professionals from multiple agencies to plan services collaboratively with the family, the mental health system, the school, and other relevant agencies. Emphasis in recent years has been focused on early childhood mental health initiatives and on broadening the concept of "systems of care" to include other populations including those who have been maltreated (Child Welfare Information Gateway, 2008).

Maternal and Child Health Services Block Grant

In 1981, the Maternal and Child Health Services Block Grant was passed. This legislation, which united seven former categorical programs into a single program, focuses on the comprehensive health and physical, psychological, and social well-being of mothers and children (Maternal and Child Health Bureau, 2000). Its goals include the establishment of a comprehensive, family-centered, community-based, coordinated system of care for children with special health care needs. Of the federal funds that are allocated for state block grants, individual states must use at least 30 percent for children with special health care needs in the achievement of this goal (Davis, 2002). In addition, the development of integrated service delivery systems are also a priority of the Bureau's Community Integrated Service System (CISS) discretionary funding program, which seeks to improve the health of mothers and children through the development and expansion of integrated health, education, and social services at the community level (Roberts & Wasik, 1996). One such effort is the State Early Childhood Comprehensive Systems Initiative (ECCS; Early Childhood Comprehensive Systems Initiative, n.d.), which fosters state planning, development, and implementation of cross-agency partnerships designed to ensure that families and communities are supported in their efforts to foster the development of children who are healthy and ready to learn when they enter school. Family support centers, which provide a range of services for vulnerable families in community contexts, usually in a single location, also receive funding under this legislation.

DEFINING THE TERMINOLOGY

The nature of collaborative terminology across service boundaries has changed over the years. In general, "interagency" or "interdisciplinary" collaboration, which tends to operate at the local or program level, has given way to such terms as "service integration" (Knitzer, 1997), "systems of care" (Child Welfare Information Gateway, 2008), and "integrated service systems" (Epps & Jackson, 2000)—terms that all envision broader systemic reform and change. Whatever the specific terminology used or level of focus, the underlying purpose is to build "partnerships to create a broad, integrated process for meeting families' multiple needs" (Child Welfare Information Gateway, 2008, p. 1). In essence it means that representatives from multiple agencies and organizations meet to identify a goal for meeting the needs of children and families that would not be achievable by any one agency and they then continue to work together to achieve the common goal (Bruner, 1991).

For this to occur, change must take place at the program and system levels of multiple service systems involved in the delivery of services to young children and their families. Many (Child Welfare Information Gateway, 2008; Knitzer, 1997; Pires, 2008) have identified basic concepts that underlie the initiatives to reform service delivery in all service sectors. Although these differ somewhat by author and/or nature of the systems being reformed, the five identified by Knitzer (1997) appear to be common to most:

Strong emphasis on family: Paramount to service integration is the delivery of family-centered services; that is, the involvement of families as partners at all levels of service delivery. Families are the primary decision makers for their children, and not simply the passive recipients of professional advice. Services are designed to meet the needs that families themselves identify. Families are viewed as capable and responsible for the care of their children. The emphasis on family also includes the participation of family members (i.e., those who represent the clientele served) in the planning and development of agency services and cross-agency/systems collaborations. This might include participation on advisory committees and task forces as well as involvement in professional development and other training activities that are sponsored by service providers.

Dedication to cultural competence: The emphasis on family includes the recognition that families are uniquely shaped by their cultural behaviors, beliefs, values, and traditions. As the demographic of the country changes, it becomes increasingly imperative that services honor and respect the cultural diversity of the families being served. Cultural values influence the services needed by a family and how, where, and when the services are delivered. Services that acknowledge cultural differences and respond accordingly are more likely to be effective. Cross-cultural competence requires that service providers understand how their own cultural backgrounds have shaped their beliefs, values, and behaviors. In turn, service providers can better serve those whose values differ.

Engagement in cross-systems collaboration: Meeting the multiple needs of children and families requires collaboration among all the services that a child and family receive. In addition, a true systems approach goes far beyond those agencies that serve a child and family directly to include the full range of potential service providers as well as those who may provide other forms of support, such as local businesses, advocacy organizations, community social groups, churches and other places of worship, and colleges and universities (Child Welfare Information Gateway, 2008).

Delivery of neighborhood and community-based services: The strengths-based-approach focus on families extends to the neighborhoods and communities in which families live. Formal and informal services and supports are available within neighborhoods and communities to help families establish, maintain, and/or strengthen the bond with other family members, friends, school and religious personnel, and others who surround them. Such community-based services also highlight the responsibility of the community/neighborhood for the welfare of its own residents.

Commitment to outcomes-based accountability: All of the defining characteristics above would be meaningless if there were no way to link modifications in service delivery to the positive outcomes of children and families. Accountability refers to the identification of expected child and family outcomes, continuous measurement of whether these benchmarks are being met, and the subsequent actions taken to modify services to better achieve outcomes. The allocation of financial resources, whether public or private, is increasingly dependent upon the measured effectiveness of the services being offered.

BENEFITS TO CROSS-SYSTEMS COLLABORATION

A variety of benefits have been identified as potential outcomes to cross-systems collaboration. Although there has been an emphasis on cross-systems and interagency collaboration since the 1980s, actual measurement of outcomes is still in its infancy (Sloper, 2004; Leslie et al., 2005). The presumed benefits discussed below provide a strong rationale for engaging in such efforts.

Improves services for children and families: The most obvious benefit to collaborative relationships among service entities is improvement in services to children and their families. Traditional service delivery tends to isolate children's needs to the area for which the service provider is responsible, often ignoring the interrelated nature of the various domains of child development. Collaborative efforts, on the other hand, recognize that the various domains of child development are integrated, and that they cannot be separated from the various domains of a child's life.

Traditional services tend to place families as passive recipients of service delivery for their children. Children interact therapeutically with professionals who are the experts, and parents receive reports of child progress. On the other hand, family-centered services recognize that the family is at the center of a child's life, that families are the decision makers for their children, and that the needs of a child must be considered within the needs of the family as a whole (Allen & Petr, 1996; Shelton & Stepanek, 1994). Although services for young children with disabilities can be family-centered without needing to entail collaborative relationships across service boundaries, once a service provider commits to family-centered service delivery, the impetus for collaboration to better meet the needs of the family whose child is receiving services from multiple entities easily becomes apparent.

Avoids costly service duplication and identifies service gaps: For families, the absence of coordination among services often means duplicative and more interactions with more professionals. More services are not necessarily better, and as we have seen in the case example, duplicated services can often be contradictory. A study by Nolan, Young, Herbert, and Wilding (2005), for example, found that children with special health care needs were receiving care coordination from more than one system. Such duplication of services usually means less efficient use of public funds. Looking broadly at the services a community provides through its various agencies (a systems perspective) not only identifies the agencies that deliver the same or similar services, but also highlights the kinds of services that are not being provided.

Reduces service inequities: All too often, the quantity and the quality of the services children receive are dependent upon the resources that their families possess. Early intervention services, for example, are used more frequently by middle-class and upper middle-class families (Kochanek & Buka, 1998; Mahoney & Filer, 1996; Sontag & Schacht, 1994). The socioeconomic class of the family, their geographic location, their ability to advocate for themselves, and their connections with others in the community are factors that influence service utilization (Zero to Three, 2009). A coordinated system of services designed to support all young children and families levels the playing field so that equal access is guaranteed to all (Zero to Three, 2009).

Facilitates an inclusive society: The neighborhoods and communities that we live in are becoming increasingly diverse—a mix of cultures and races, languages, economic levels, sexual orientations, and religions. The delivery of services in neighborhood and community settings helps to insure that young children with disabilities become an integral part of these diverse communities and that they remain a part of those communities as they grow into adulthood, obviously adding a further dimension to the existing diversity. Traditional services, which may be provided in centers separate from nondisabled peers or in neighborhoods distant from those in which they live, tend to isolate children with disabilities from their neighborhoods and communities. Connections made in child care centers and local programs and organizations strengthen the overall bond and support among neighbors, hopefully providing avenues from more informal supports.

Ensures positive outcomes and avoids school failure: A coordinated system of services across health care, education, and social services is intended to provide all families with the supports they need so that their children receive an excellent start in life and develop the foundation to succeed once they reach school age. Children experiencing multiple risks such as homelessness, child abuse, birth abnormalities, inadequate health care, low-quality schools, and violence are at significant risk for school failure; and addressing these factors falls outside of the authority of public education, requiring collaboration among multiple service providers (Rouse & Fantuzzo, 2009).

ACHIEVING INTERAGENCY COLLABORATION

Facilitators and Barriers

Achieving collaboration within an organization is never easy, so achieving collaboration not only across agencies but also across service sectors is ever more daunting. Both facilitators of and barriers to the success of interagency collaboration have been identified in the literature. A study of departments and social agencies in Ohio, for example, identified the facilitators of collaboration as falling into three primary categories: commitment, strong leadership, and communication (Johnson, Zorn, Kai Yung Tam, LaMontagne, & Johnson, 2003). Similar results were obtained by Sloper (2004) in review of the literature relating to the coordination of children's and family's services in England. A solid commitment to the effort must be demonstrated at all levels of the agencies involved and requires that key decision makers in each agency be willing to make the necessary adjustments within their agencies to further the joint goals of the collaboration. A multiagency steering committee made up of individuals who can commit resources to the joint effort helps to ensure the effort's success. Additionally, good systems of communication and information sharing across agencies, including the use of information technology, are necessary as the work of the group progresses. Other facilitating factors that were found to relate to the joint work of the interagency group include the development of clear goals for the collaborative endeavor and the specification of roles and responsibilities with explicit timetables for carrying out the tasks involved. Appropriate support and training for staff on how to work together in new ways also lends itself to facilitating successful collaboration.

It is clear that the relationships among individuals involved in the collaboration can influence the effectiveness of the endeavor. Mutual mistrust of workers from other agencies can undermine joint efforts (Darlington, Feeney, & Rixon, 2005). Respect for the work of other agencies, the disciplines involved in that work, and the workers themselves are fundamental to the success of joint collaboration (Darlington et al., 2005; Johnson et al., 2003). Differences in professional ideologies and agency cultures (Sloper, 2004) as well as disciplinary knowledge domains and boundaries (Darlington et al., 2005), often referred to as "turf issues" (Johnson et al., 2003), can contribute to an atmosphere of mistrust. Unrealistic expectations of what other agencies or disciplines do can further contribute to fundamental mistrust. There is some empirical evidence, however, that interprofessional development and training help to breakdown some of these barriers to working collaboratively (Sloper, 2004). Such occasions may serve to fill in some of the information gaps that professionals have about the roles of other agencies and their workers and to begin to reduce some of the misperceptions that exist across agency boundaries.

Constant reorganization of agencies, financial uncertainty within agencies, frequent staff turnover, and the absence of qualified staff (Sloper, 2004) are among the barriers to cross-agency collaboration. Inadequate allocation of resources, such as lack of time, heavy workloads, and lack of appropriate community resources, can also undermine the achievement of joint interagency goals (Darlington et al, 2005). Laws and regulations relating to confidentiality can limit cross-agency communication about service integration for a specific child or family (Darlington et al. 2005).

Developing a Vision

Specific cross-agency collaborations, whether at the local or state level, require that the parties involved devote time to developing a joint vision of what they expect to transpire. Many of our national professional organizations, policy centers, and foundations, either individually or jointly, have published position statements and white papers to fuel these state and local efforts. These efforts also serve as a way of supporting and motivating service providers within specific disciplines to loosen the boundaries of their own professional cultures to include greater collaborative efforts. Some states, such as Vermont, have also developed detailed vision statements. Several examples are provided below.

American Academy of Pediatrics

The American Academy of Pediatrics (AAP) takes an active role in developing policy statements around a large variety of critical topics delineating the role of pediatricians and pediatric primary care. For example, since the early 1990s with the proposal of the concept of a medical home, it has set forth the standard that all children should have accessible, continuous, comprehensive, family-centered, coordinated, compassionate, and culturally effective medical care (American Academy of Pediatrics, 2002). Within the medical home, the role of the pediatric health care professional includes surveillance and screening of infants for disabilities and delays in development, referral to early intervention services and necessary medical etiologic diagnostic evaluations, collaborating in the development of Individual Education Programs (IEPs) and Individualized Family Service Plans (IFSPs) if a child is eligible for early intervention services, and supporting families in their efforts to secure and maintain services for their children with disabilities (American Academy of Pediatrics, 2007). Furthermore, the AAP offers a policy that includes an algorithm for developmental surveillance and screening within the pediatric medical home (American Academy of Pediatrics, 2006). Another policy statement has proposed that the medical home of a child with special health care needs is an ideal setting for identifying, referring, and coordinating the services a child receives in the health, education, and other community programs (American Academy of Pediatrics, 2005).

DEC and NAEYC

In April 2009, the Division for Early Childhood of the Council for Exceptional Children (DEC) and the National Association for the Education of Young Children (NAEYC) jointly published a position paper on early childhood inclusion that sets forth a definition and vision. The statement recognizes that it is "the right of every infant and young child and his or her family, regardless of ability, to participate in a broad range of activities and contexts as full members of families, communities, and society" (DEC/NAEYC, 2009, p. 1) and that the achievement of quality early childhood inclusion requires collaboration among key stakeholders (e.g., families, practitioners, specialists, administrators). It calls upon these key stakeholders to develop an "infrastructure of systems-level supports" to include "multiple opportunities for communication and collaboration" among groups, specialized services and therapies that are "implemented in a coordinated fashion and integrated with general early care and education services," and "funding policies that promote the pooling of resources." Among the strategies for achieving high-quality early childhood inclusion is the development of an integrated professional development system.

National Institute for Health Care Management Foundation (NIHCM)

The NIHCM is a nonprofit, nonpartisan organization dedicated to improving the effectiveness, efficiency, and quality of America's health care system. In August 2009, it published an overview describing strategies that support the integration of mental health into pediatric primary care based on advances in research and policy trends. The publication elucidates a rationale and a vision of "coordinated, seamless care that supports emotional well-being" (National Institute for Health Care Management, 2009, p. 2) in which there is collaboration among the private and public health and mental health sectors. Numerous examples of such collaborations are provided throughout the document.

State of Vermont

In 2005, the state of Vermont developed and published a state-level agreement intended to "ensure, guide, and monitor coordination and collaboration" (Vermont Agency of Human Services, 2005, p. 1) among Early Care, Health, and Education Programs and agencies. The agreement (Vermont Agency of Human Services, 2005) developed by 10 service entities, provides guidance for developing interagency agreements at the state, regional, and local levels. The document sets forth a vision that describes shared responsibilities across programs and agencies that are working in partnership with each other to serve young children with disabilities and their families. A set of principles, which includes such terms as family-centered, universally designed system, equitable, and inclusive, are defined. These principles are then applied to a set of agreed-upon practices (e.g., outreach/screening, referrals, initial evaluations, development and implementation of child and family plans, transportation) that all agencies and programs that work in partnership with each other will attempt to operationalize in their selected shared activities. For example, the section on Outreach states that all involved will:

1. Understand and share information about available services and resources
2. Inform families about early care, health and education services, and resources in their communities
3. Promote public awareness of all community resources available to children and families
4. Ensure that families have access to information about health insurance including Medicaid and EPSDT (Vermont Agency of Human Services, 2005, p. 5)

The Process of Collaboration

Obviously, collaboration is not an end in itself; rather the focus is on creating changes within and across programs, agencies, and systems that better support children with disabilities and their families. To this end, we must see the process of collaboration as central to the much broader concept known as "systems change." Systems change can be defined as "change efforts that strive to shift the underlying infrastructure within a community or targeted context to support a desired outcome, including shifting existing policies and practices, resource allocations, relational structures, community norms and values, and skills and attitudes" (Foster-Fishman & Behrens, 2007, p. 191). Fields such as business, social work, and psychology have all been engaged in studying systems change to determine not only how change occurs and how best to achieve it, but also to develop theories that enhance our understanding of the phenomenon independent of the systems marked for change or the goals identified.

Cummings and Worley (as cited in Epps & Jackson, 2000) describe a model for the change consisting of five major activities: (1) motivating change, (2) creating a vision, (3) developing political support, (4) managing the transition, and (5) sustaining momentum. Epps and Jackson (2000) apply this framework to developing integrated and collaborative systems of early intervention services. They explain how the motivation for change emerges from current dissatisfaction with services and exposure to new ideas and practices. The tension between the two creates the motivation for change and sets the stage for the development of a shared vision for change to include a mission statement and outcomes among the agencies and programs involved. Change cannot be accomplished without the active involvement of all the key stakeholders, including families, and the development of external political support for the change. All stakeholders work together in an atmosphere of commitment to plan the activities that are intended to accomplish the reform in services and to execute them accordingly, first as a pilot with corrective actions as needed and then eventually developing and sustaining the momentum to implement on a larger scale. Momentum is sustained by providing the necessary resources and supporting the agents of change by assisting them in developing new competencies and skills and reinforcing their new behaviors. Additionally, the process is cyclical, so that as change is accomplished, the parties strive to continue to identify areas of dissatisfaction that would warrant continued change efforts.

Foster-Fishman, Nowell, and Yang (2007) describe a dynamic approach to systems change in human services that is based upon Soft Systems Methodologies (Checkland, 1981) and Systems Dynamic Thinking (Forrester, 1969). They hypothesize that many systems-change efforts do not achieve the level of outcome that is anticipated because the systemic nature of the contexts involved and the complexity of the change process are ignored. They propose a four-step process for transformative systems change: (1) bounding the system, (2) understanding fundamental system parts as potential root causes, (3) assessing system interactions, and (4) identifying levers for change. Bounding the system entails identifying the stakeholders who then engage in a dialogic process to define the problem, acknowledging as part of Soft Systems Methodologies that different stakeholders, because they have different worldviews, will perceive both the problem and the potential solutions differently. Once the problem has been adequately negotiated among all the parties, the "system" is defined or bounded. This will entail identifying the system levels, programs, organizations, and consumers relevant to the issue. The process of understanding the relevant systems parts requires stakeholders to identify system norms, resources, regulations, and operations that maintain the system's current existence. Such efforts include both the apparent system as well as the "below the surface" attitudes, values, and beliefs of the individuals who work in the system. Exploring these from the perspectives of different levels, programs, organizations, and consumers will assist in identifying potential areas of support or resistance. The assessment of systems interactions provides opportunities for stakeholders to determine how the parts of the system interact with each other so as to identify how interaction patterns need to change for the shared goal to be accomplished. This in-depth study of the system will then permit the identification of strategic levers for bringing about the changes in the system.

Charles Bruner (2004) developed a Theory of Change for the Build Initiative, a multi-state, multi-foundation effort focused on young children and their development to help the participating states to "build a coordinated system of programs, policies, and services—an early learning system—that is responsive to the needs of families, careful in the use of private and public resources and effective in preparing our youngest children for a successful future" (Build Initiative, 2005, p. 1). The Build Initiative embodies three theories of change analogous to the development and implementation of a complex construction project. The first theory recognizes that a master plan must be developed. There are many components to an early learning system, which must be identified. The "system" to be developed must be defined, and the goals of the system must be agreed upon by the people involved. The Build Initiative has identified four components to a state-level early learning system: (1) health and nutrition, (2) early care and education, (3) family support, and (4) special needs/early intervention. The second theory, which focuses on the critical strategies needed to build a state early learning system, consists of eight critical elements. The groundwork consists of the recognition of the need and the development of a shared early learning vision (Elements 1 and 2) with the support of political leadership from the governor and state legislature (Element 3). Implementation is carried out by the capacity and expertise of midlevel managers (Element 4) to develop programs, actions, and policy successes (Element 5). Momentum is built politically to develop and maintain the system by public awareness and support (Element 6), and mobilization and advocacy from outside the government sector to support the changes (Element 7). Capacity is built by the alignment of multiple factors (Element 8) typically focusing attention on several new initiatives and/or policy changes per year. The third theory of change relates to the catalytic role that the Build Initiative has in supporting the states in constructing their early learning systems. Through the technical assistance provided by the Build Initiative, including evaluation to provide essential continuous improvement and development, states identified to benefit from this "inertia-breaking final investment" (Bruner, 2004, p. 11) have been able to move substantially forward in developing an early learning system. These states are Illinois, Michigan, Minnesota, New Jersey, New York, Ohio, Pennsylvania, and Washington.

Functions of Collaborative Models

Systems reform requires significant effort on the part of the agencies involved. Rather than tackling an overhaul of the total system of services all at once, it is often productive to focus collaborations on one area or to develop a plan in which each service function is modified sequentially. Typically these functions might include the following:

Child Find and Screening

Child find and screening refers to the process of identifying a population of children who are in need of further assessment. Traditionally, each early intervention agency in a community might have its own processes and procedures for executing child find and screening. However, agencies might collaborate with one another to develop joint public-service campaigns that educate the general population about disabilities or other risk factors. They also may sponsor joint opportunities for families to bring their children for a more formal assessment of health and developmental risks, referring children as necessary for in-depth evaluations to the appropriate agencies. Collaboration reduces duplication of services, saving taxpayer dollars in the public service campaigns, and may serve families better because screening and referral for evaluation are likely to be more comprehensive.

Primary medical care can also play an important role in child find, screening, and referral for more in-depth assessment and, as appropriate, treatment (National Institute for Health Care Management, 2009). Pediatricians, family practitioners, and other medical professionals who see children for routine care are well positioned to screen for mental health (National Institute for Health Care Management, 2009) and other types of disorders (American Academy of Pediatrics, 2006). Such an approach requires greater coordination and collaboration of primary care physicians with community service providers so as to promote the development of a seamless system of care for both physical and mental health needs. The National Institute for Health Care Management (2009), for example, has proposed three models for the integration of mental health into pediatric primary care: (1) consultation in which primary care providers, particularly in rural areas, consult with child psychiatrists in other locations; (2) co-location of mental health special-ists within the practice itself to facilitate treatment planning and refer-ral; and (3) collaboration in which primary care providers using the medical home model establish partnerships with community mental health care providers. Real-life examples of each model type are pro-vided within their report.

Assessment

Assessment encompasses in-depth evaluation for the purpose of determining the need for early intervention services. Traditionally, every service agency develops and executes its own process for assess-ment following the regulations set forth by the service entity. A col-laborative focus on assessment might include agreement on a core of assessment tools that might be used to determine service eligibility or cross-agency acceptance of assessment results for a child or family to limit the number of assessments a child or family must endure.

Service Coordination

Service coordination refers to the function of assisting families to nego-tiate the range of services that might be available to them within the community. Although some systems and agencies may offer these services to families, others may not. Typically, service coordination for families is a within-system function, so a family may have a service coordinator for health services and another for educational services. Collaboration across service sectors would make it possible to stream-line the service coordination function. For example, both health and educational services might be negotiated by a single service co-ordinator, thus reducing the possibility of service duplication and con-tradictory services. It also reduces the number of professionals with whom a family must interact.

Intervention

Usually each service provider develops their own plan of services for a young child with disabilities and his or her family. Interventions take place in locations according to the requirements of the individualized plan and the regulations governing the system or agency in which the services are offered. Collaborations across agencies might involve the development of a single individualized service plan in which the roles and responsibilities of the professionals of each agency are carefully identified, resolving any obvious differences in approach. Services might take place in one or more locations that are determined to be convenient for the family (e.g., child care). The coordination of interventions also assists a family and the professionals involved to grasp more easily the full range of services and how they relate to one another. Jointly collecting and sharing progress data can provide the basis for empirically based program modifications for a given child.

Professional Development

Professional development refers to the provision of in-service educational experiences and training that are provided to professionals within an agency or service system. Generally speaking, every agency or service system has its own agenda for professional development. Additionally, professionals may also have continuing educational requirements to fulfill to maintain professional licensure. Collaboration across agencies and systems might involve joint planning of professional development opportunities in a community or service sector so that professionals from multiple agencies can participate. These opportunities for professionals from other agencies to meet each other not only assist in breaking down some of the cultural and attitudinal barriers to cross-agency collaboration, but they can also set the stage for jointly learning new patterns of professional behavior that support collaborative efforts.

Proposed Comprehensive Models

Comprehensive models of systems change focus on the development of the full range of services for a specified population of children and families. The Build Initiative described earlier to develop statewide early learning systems represents one comprehensive model of services for young children. Examples of two additional proposed models are described below.

The Zero to Three Model

Zero to Three, an interdisciplinary organization devoted to the welfare of our youngest citizens, recently proposed a comprehensive model of services for all infants and toddlers (Zero to Three, 2009). The model encompasses services from the three major systems: (1) physical and mental health services, (2) family support services, and (3) early care and education. According to the model, physical and mental health services include health insurance coverage, prenatal care, primary and preventative care, guidance for parents to support healthy child development, and developmental screenings. Family support services include parenting education, family basic economic support, supportive work and family policies (e.g., paid family leave), and special supports for families in crisis. Early care and education includes quality child care in a variety of settings, Early Head Start, and early intervention for children with disabilities. This community-based comprehensive coordinated system of services includes seven essential components: (1) governance and leadership, (2) quality improvement, (3) accountability and evaluation, (4) financing, (5) public engagement and political will building, (6) regulations and standards, and (7) professional development.

Foster Care Model

Leslie et al. (2005) describes a comprehensive model for health, developmental, and mental health professionals to collaborate with child welfare to better serve children in foster care. Children in foster care often have significant developmental and mental health issues (Sedlak & Boadhurst, 1996; Szilagyi, 2009) that lead to school failure and as they grow older, high rates of dropping out of school and delinquency (Cohen et al., 1998; Newton, Litrownik, & Landsverk, 2000; Smucker, Kauffman, & Ball, 1996; Taussig, 2002; Zima et al., 2000). Studies have estimated that the prevalence of developmental disabilities among those in foster care to be as high as 60 percent, in contrast to the general population with estimates of 4–10 percent (Leslie et al., 2005). The framework that Leslie and colleagues describe is based on a study of promising practices in meeting the physical, mental, and developmental needs of young children in foster care (Woolverton, 2002). Eleven components were identified through telephone interviews and site visits to nine programs that together provide a framework for a comprehensive approach to addressing the needs of children in foster care: (1) initial screening and comprehensive health assessment, (2) access to health care service and treatment, (3) management of health care data and information, (4) coordination of care, (5) collaboration among systems, (6) family participation, (7) attention to cultural issues, (8) monitoring and evaluation, (9) training/education, (10) funding strategies, and (11) designing managed care to fit the needs of children in the child welfare system. Although no one program in the study contained all 11 components, taken together, the list identifies the critical components of a model program.

Toolkits and Guidelines

Many projects have been funded in various human service sectors that have focused on the implementation of the cross-agency collaboration and systems reform due to the wide range of legislation described earlier. Many projects have developed toolkits and guidelines that might be helpful to other programs pursuing similar goals. Technical assistance agencies and some states also have published materials. A wealth of such information is available on the Internet. A few of these sites are highlighted here.

Champions for Inclusive Communities

Champions for Inclusion Communities is a "national center designed to support communities in organizing services for families of children and youth with special health care needs" (Champions for Inclusive Communities, n.d.). This organization is devoted to providing assistance in the development of systems of care for this population. There are six national centers, each committed to a different system of care performance indicator: (1) Families as Partners, (2) Access to Medical Home, (3) Early and Continuous Screening, (4) Adequate Insurance, (5) Organized Services, and (6) Transition to Adulthood. Numerous resources are offered to support the development of these measureable indicators, including the identification of "Star Communities" recognized for their implementation of community-based service systems.

Bright Futures

Bright Futures is a national health promotion initiative that was originally begun by the Maternal and Child Health Bureau in 1990. It is now currently administrated by the American Academy of Pediatrics in conjunction with state and federal Bright Futures projects. The initiative is dedicated to the "principle that every child deserves to be healthy and that optimal health involves a trusting relationship between the health professional, the child, the family, and the community as partners in health practice" (National Center for Education in

Maternal and Child Health, Georgetown University, 2008, p. 1). Information and training materials are available on the Web site to assist pediatricians and others to implement systems-of-care principles across agencies in the implementation of a community-based approach to mental health services.

Head Start

The Head Start Web site provides ample resources designed to assist Head Start programs in the development of community partnerships (Early Childhood Learning and Knowledge Center, n.d.). The guide on the collaborative process (Early Childhood Learning and Knowledge Center, 2000), for example, identifies a five-step process: (1) getting together, (2) building trust and ownership, (3) strategic planning, (4) taking action, and (5) evaluation. These steps, which are elucidated on the Web site, capture many of the collaborative principles described in other portions of this chapter.

SUCCESSFUL COLLABORATIONS: THE EVIDENCE BASE

Although legislative mandates for cross-agency and cross-system collaboration have been in existence since the 1980s for a range of populations, the evidence base available measuring the outcomes for children, youth, and their families is very slim (Leslie et al., 2005; Sloper, 2004). Most of the published information has focused on descriptions of collaborations, processes, and changes to service delivery, some of which have been referenced earlier in this chapter. Such information is plentiful and can be found in peer-reviewed journal articles, reports of projects and initiatives supported by government and other funders, and Internet sites of specific projects, technical assistance providers, and government agencies. The few studies that have examined actual outcomes for children and their families have generally focused on older children with emotional and behavioral disorders; little outcome data are currently available for evaluating the effectiveness for young children and their families.

Modifications to Service Delivery

A critical first step in understanding how collaborative initiatives are transforming service delivery across the country is empirical documentation of both the processes used to change service delivery and the manner and extent to which services have been changed.

Reports

Initiatives devoted to the development of early learning systems for young children have published reports of the types of modifications that have taken place in participating states.

The first evaluation report of the Early Childhood Comprehensive Systems Grant Program of the Maternal and Child Health Bureau (Lewin Group, 2007) investigated the progress of the 2005 cohort of 20 states receiving funding. Through a survey of participants, findings reported include increased enrollment in public health insurance programs for children, increased mental health trainings for early childhood providers, improved quality of child care, increased awareness of the importance of parent education, and increased quality of family support programs.

In the evaluation of the Build Initiative from 2002 to 2009 (Bruner & Wright, 2009) there is a chart documenting the changes in the seven participating states. Accomplishments that most directly relate to children with disabilities and the goals of this chapter include expanded health coverage and expanded early intervention services for children with disabilities in five states; expanded developmental health and child mental screening, services, and training in six states; improved integrated planning and actions across systems in all seven states; and improved and expanded family support and parent education in six states. The chart also underscores important achievements in the political, governance, and leadership arenas that are necessary in sustaining and further developing state early childhood systems.

The U.S. Office of Head Start (2007) published a report consisting of state profiles that summarize each state's collaboration efforts. State reports are organized into the 10 current priority areas of health care, homelessness, welfare, child care, education, disabilities, child welfare, community literacy, community services, and professional development. The information is not aggregated across states.

Empirical Studies

Although much descriptive material is available documenting systemic changes, there are few peer-reviewed empirical studies. The studies presented below that were published in peer-reviewed journals address various types of systems modifications, although unfortunately, they are not exclusively focused on young children.

Bruns, Rast, Peterson, Walker, and Bosworth (2006) documented how data collection and analysis were used to inform statewide systems-change efforts in Nevada to provide wraparound services to children with emotional and behavioral disorders. Wraparound services represent a collaborative planning process that includes family members, natural support networks, and service providers from multiple agencies, resulting in an individual treatment plan that maintains the child in his family and community. The evaluative steps in this collaboration between the child welfare and mental health agencies included assessing the statewide need for wraparound services, evaluating a pilot wraparound program, measuring and improving program implementation, and evaluating program impact and unaddressed needs in the state.

Tebes et al. (2005) examined access to services across time in a statewide systems-of-care initiative in Rhode Island for comprehensive services to children with emotional and behavioral disorders. The investigation, which studied 2,073 children over an eight-year period, assessed the extent to which children received the services recommended by multiagency case review teams within three months of their recommendation at the beginning, middle, and end of the establishment of the system. Access to services improved across time. The study also showed that the number and variety of children and agencies involved increased over time.

Lannon et al. (2008) studied the extent to which 15 pediatric practices in nine different states adopted Bright Futures strategies to include a greater focus on mental health following nine months of collaborative learning. These pediatric practices on average increased their usage of the 21 possible Bright Futures strategies from 10 to 15. The most frequently implemented strategies were recall/reminder systems, linkages to community resources, and systematically asking parents if their children had special health care needs. The study demonstrated that the collaborative training program, involving teams from each practice of a doctor, ancillary clinical staff, and an administrative representative, resulted in modifications to pediatric practice.

Several studies point to increased developmental and mental health screening and referral by pediatric practices. We have evidence that children referred to mental health services by their pediatricians are more likely to actually receive those services (Lavigne et al., 1998). Pediatric residents who received training about developmental screening and community referral improved their knowledge regarding these topics (Bauer, Smith, Chien, Berry, & Msall, 2009). One year later, chart audits demonstrated increased use of screening tools and more referrals to community services. A project in North Carolina to establish developmental screening within well-child pediatric visits demonstrated increased screening rates over a two-year period (Earls, Andrews, & Hay, 2009). Physicians were more likely to screen younger children than older children and more likely to refer children to early intervention and other community programs for developmental rather than behavioral concerns of parents.

Measurement of Child and Family Outcomes

One source of evidence supporting positive outcomes for more collaborative cross-systems service delivery is the National Evaluation of the Comprehensive Community Mental Health Services for Children and their Families Program (Center for Mental Health Services, 2003). The evaluation collected and analyzed data from the implementation of the program from 1997 to 2000. Of the 11,814 children who served in the program, more than half were over 12 years of age. Results revealed that children's behavioral and emotional strengths increased, improved school performance was related to improvements in behavioral and emotional problems, and most children received services in community settings rather than in restrictive placements. In a comparison with matched non-systems-of-care communities, the systems-of-care communities were determined to have scored higher on the application of systems-of-care principles and were more family-focused. Greater clinically significant change was also demonstrated from intake to 12 months in the systems-of-care communities (Stephens et al., 2005; Stephens, Holden, & Hernandez, 2004).

Several studies have documented the pre-referral factors (e.g., demographic characteristics, referral) that predict better outcomes in a systems-of-care approach. Anderson, Effland, Kooreman, and Wright (2006) examined data from the Dawn Program in Indiana for youth with DSM IV or special education diagnoses. Results of the study demonstrated that age was the only predictor of outcome, with younger children having better outcomes than older children within the first six months of services. Walrath, Ybarra, and Holdern (2006), using data from the Comprehensive Community Mental Health Services for Children Program, revealed that children with more severe indicators of impairment (i.e., higher levels of functional impairment, higher levels of caregiver strain, and poorer academic functioning) were more likely to improve within the first six months in the system. However, minority racial/ethnic background, out-of-home placement, and history of substance abuse were factors that predicted deterioration within the same time period. Using data from the National Survey of Child and Adolescent Well-Being, Hurlburt et al. (2004) examined mental health service usage among 2,823 child welfare cases in 97 counties across the United States. Results indicated that increased coordination between child welfare and mental health agencies reduced the disparities between mental health service usage among white and African American children.

Horwitz, Owens, and Simms (2000) compared children entering foster care who had received a comprehensive multidisciplinary program with those who had received traditional services. The two groups had comparable medical, educational, developmental, and mental health problems, but children in the comprehensive program were more likely to be referred for developmental, mental health, and medical health services by their providers than those receiving customary services.

EMERGING TRENDS AND NEEDS

This chapter has provided an overview of the goals, benefits and challenges, strategies, and effectiveness of crossing agency and systems boundaries in the delivery of services to young children with disabilities and their families. Young children with disabilities and their families are often involved in multiple service-delivery systems in the domains of health care, education, and social services. The involvement of multiple professionals from multiple systems not only complicates the lives of families, but also may not be the most effective or efficient use of services for children. Integrated services systems are more likely to better serve the needs of children and families and to use the dollars available more efficiently.

Federal legislation in the areas of health and human services and education have responded to this need by calling for system reforms that are family-centered, culturally competent, collaborative across agencies and systems, community-based, and accountable. Government and foundation grants since the 1980s have funded such systems of care primarily in the areas of mental health and child welfare for children over 5 years of age, adolescents, and their families.

More recently, the emphasis has been on the development of early childhood systems that integrate health care, early care and education, early intervention including mental health, and family education and support.

Systems change can take place at the local, regional, or state level and can involve as few as two agencies or the majority, if not all the agencies, in a given community. The potential benefits include, first and foremost, improvements in services to children and families. Modifications in service delivery have been well documented in all sectors, including the practices of pediatricians (e.g., Bauer et al., 2009; Earls et al., 2009; Lannon et al., 2008), mental health services for children (e.g., Bruns et al., 2006; Center for Mental Health Services, 2003; Tebes et al., 2005), children in foster care (e.g., Horwitz et al., 2000), and young children generally (e.g., Bruner & Wright, 2009; Office of Head Start, 2007). A change in services is not necessarily an improvement in services. Although accountability is emphasized as one of the hallmarks of the systems-of-care approach, relatively little information is available, apart from the Comprehensive Mental Health Service Program (Center for Mental Health Services, 2003) documenting modifications in child and family outcomes. More studies in general are needed to demonstrate the comparative effectiveness of a systems-of-care approach over more traditional services and, in particular, there needs to be a specific focus on children under age 5 and their families.

Other presumed benefits also are supported by very little empirical evidence. These include the avoidance of costly service duplication; a reduction in service inequities, for which there is some evidence (Hurlburt et al., 2004); and the facilitation of an inclusive society, a benefit that can be documented perhaps by fewer out-of-home and restrictive placements (Center for Mental Health Services, 2003). More careful study is needed in these areas as well with an emphasis on young children, particularly those with disabilities.

On the other hand, theories of change, and especially the technology to bring about family-centered, culturally competent, community-based systems of services through interagency and intersystem collaboration, are widely available. The facilitators and inhibitors of interagency and cross-system collaboration are well-documented. In addition to the mandates of the federal government, professional organizations, policy institutes, and technical assistance agencies have assisted in furthering the development of the vision for collaboration and systems reform. The steps involved may be conceptualized differently for different collaborative efforts, but they almost always involve a common under-standing of need among agencies, the development of a joint vision and joint goals, the development and implementation of a strategic plan, and the collection of data to assist in the developmental efforts and to measure effectiveness. Consumers themselves must play an inte-gral role in these developmental efforts to ensure that the services devel-oped serve the needs of children and families. The technology that is available on Web sites and in other published documents focuses heavily on the initial steps in this process. The technology that assists agencies in the collection and use of data for formative and summative evaluation of the efforts, however, deserves to be better developed.

CROSSING THE COUNTY LINE: THE PRESBYLSKI FAMILY

To address the needs of the Presbylski family, two interagency solu-tions seem apparent—that the early intervention program in Monroe County provide services to Carrie in her Smithfield County child care program, or that Smithfield County provide early intervention serv-ices to Carrie with the assumption that Monroe County compensate them for these efforts. A meeting between the two local early interven-tion administrators in Monroe and Smithfield counties and Mr. and Mrs. Presbylski resulted in an interagency agreement in which the par-ties decided that the best solution would be for Carrie's current teacher to go to the ABC Child Care Center located only a mile from the Presbylski home. This logistically simple solution would preserve continuity of services for both Carrie and her family with minimal administrative modification.

WHO TO BELIEVE: THE GARZA FAMILY

The solution for the Garza family could be addressed at either the local or state level. At the local level, a meeting of the two agencies and the family could be held. The relevant personnel from the early interven-tion agency would include the home-based teacher, the speech-language pathologist, and a program administrator. The therapeutic staff support supervisor would represent the Behavioral Health Agency, since she is responsible for the design and implementation of Paco's program. The meeting should focus on resolving the issues around the nature of Paco's communication program (whether it should be picture- or sign-based) and the role of the parents in implementing the intervention. This will probably require the modification of the treatment plans for each agency and a clarification of the roles of each agency in the implementation of the agreed-upon approach to Paco's communication programming. In accordance with the provision of family-centered services, Paco's parents would be partners in making any decisions. In addition, a plan for communication among service providers might include scheduling periodic meetings and some form of regular communication between direct service providers (perhaps a log that is kept in the home) to communicate activities, progress, and issues that may arise. Financing the joint planning meetings will be an issue that both agencies will need to contemplate. However, since both agencies support periodic meetings with parents as part of their regulatory procedures, the joint scheduling of such meetings could be easily accomplished.

An alternative local solution would be recognition by both agencies that many children receiving early intervention services also receive behavioral health services. The two local authorities could engage themselves in a local systems-change effort to jointly develop a standard set of procedures to be used in such cases. Such efforts would require the agencies to define the need; develop a set of goals/objectives for the collaboration; involve all the relevant stakeholders, including families; develop the procedures; field test the procedures in a pilot run followed by evaluation of the outcomes and adjustment of the procedures; build capacity for these changes within the system through joint training of personnel; and evaluate both the implementation and the child and family outcomes. Many of the procedures and resources identified in this chapter would be useful in these efforts.

A state-level solution to the issues obviously requires greater systemic change. A need for change may include recognition that families statewide who are receiving services from both agencies might be better served if there were more collaboration in planning and implementing services. Such collaboration might avoid wasteful service duplications or contradictions and, consequently, unnecessary confusion for parents. It might help the state find a pathway to greater service efficiency and coherence, potentially more progress for children, and perhaps to resources that might be freed up to design new types of service configurations. For example, the development of a single program/treatment plan that meets the needs of both systems might be developed. The joint efforts of both might provide the brainpower to envision an even more innovative step in the collaboration—the development of a cross-system program for teaching parents intervention strategies to meet the needs of their young children with autism in their homes and communities. Such a program could augment the current service configuration and better empower parents to address the needs of their children.

References

Ackoff, R. L., & Rovin, S. (2003). *Redesigning society.* Stanford, CA: Stanford Business Books.

Allen, R. I., & Petr, C. G. (1996). Toward developing standards and measurements for family-centered practice in family support programs. In G. Singer, L. Powers, & A. Olson (Eds.), *Redefining family support: Innovations in public-private partnerships* (pp. 57–85). Baltimore: Paul H. Brookes.

American Academy of Pediatrics. (2002). Policy statement: The medical home. *Pediatrics, 110,* 184–186.

American Academy of Pediatrics. (2005). Policy statement: Care coordination in the medical home: Integrating health and related systems of care for children with special health care needs. *Pediatrics, 116,* 1238–1244.

American Academy of Pediatrics. (2006). Policy statement: Identifying infants and young children with developmental disorders in the medical home: An algorithm for developmental surveillance and screening. *Pediatrics, 118,* 405–420.

American Academy of Pediatrics. (2007). Policy statement: Role of the medical home in family-centered early intervention services. *Pediatrics, 120,* 1153–1158.

Anderson, J. A., Effland, V. S., Kooreman, H., & Wright, E. R. (2006). Predicting functional improvement over time in a system of care. *Families in Society: The Journal of Contemporary Social Services, 87,* 438–446.

Bauer, S. C., Smith, P. J., Chien, A. T., Berry, A. D., & Msall, M. E. (2009). Educating pediatric residents about developmental and social-emotional health. *Infants and Young Children, 22,* 309–320.

Bruner, C. (1991). *Thinking collaboratively: Ten questions and answers to help policy makers improve children's services.* Washington, DC: Education and Human Services Consortium.

Bruner, C. (2004). Toward a theory of change for the Build Initiative: A discussion paper. Retrieved from http://www.buildinitiative.org/content/about-us

Bruner, C., & Wright, M. S. (2009). The first seven years: The Build Initiative and Early Childhood Systems Development, 2002 to 2009. Retrieved from http://www.buildinitiative.org/files/BUILD%20-%20First%207%20years.pdf

Bruns, E. J., Rast, J., Peterson, C., Walker, J., & Bosworth, J. (2006). Spreadsheets, service providers, and the statehouse: Using data and the wraparound process to reform systems for children and families. *American Journal of Community Psychology, 38,* 201–212.

Build Initiative. (2005). The Build Initiative's Theory of Change. Retrieved from http://www.buildinitiative.org/content/about-us

California Department of Education. (2007). *Handbook on developing and evaluating interagency collaboration in early childhood special education programs.* Retrieved

February 12, 2010, from http://www.cde.ca.gov/sp/se/fp/documents/eciacolbrtn.pdf

Center for Mental Health Services. (2003). *Annual report to Congress 2002–2003: The Comprehensive Community Mental Health Services for Children and Their Families Program—Evaluation findings.* Retrieved from http://download.ncadi.samhsa.gov/ken/pdf/SMA03-CBE2002/CongReport20022003FINAL PUBLICATION.pdf

Champions for Inclusive Communities. (n.d.). *Welcome.* Retrieved from http://www.championsinc.org/

Checkland, P. (1981). *Systems thinking: Systems practice.* Chichester, West Sussex: Wiley.

Child Abuse Prevention and Treatment Act (P.L. 104-235). (1996). Retrieved from http://www.acf.hhs.gov/programs/cb/laws_policies/cblaws/public_law/pl104_235/pl104_235.htm

Child Welfare Information Gateway. (2008, February). *Systems of Care.* Retrieved from http://www.childwelfare.gov/pubs/soc/soc.pdf

Cohen, N. J., Menna, R., Vallance, D. D., Barwick, M. A., Im, N., & Horodezky, N. B. (1998). Language, social cognitive processing, and behavioral characteristics of psychiatrically disturbed children with previously identified and unsuspected language impairments. *Journal of Child Psychology and Psychiatry, 39,* 853–864.

Darlington, Y., Feeney, J. A., & Rixon, K. (2005). Interagency collaboration between child protection and mental health services: Practices, attitudes and barriers. *Child Abuse and Neglect, 29,* 1085–1098.

Davis, R. (2002). Maternal and Child Health Block Grant. *Encyclopedia of Public Health.* Retrieved March 11, 2010, from Encyclopedia.com: http://www.encyclopedia.com/doc/1G2-3404000524.html

Division for Early Childhood of the Council for Exceptional Children & National Association for the Education of Young Children. (2009). *Early childhood inclusion: A joint position statement of the Division for Early Childhood (DEC) and the National Association for the Education of Young Children (NAEYC).* Chapel Hill: University of North Carolina, FPG Child Development Institute. Retrieved from http://community.fpg.unc.edu/resources/articles/Early_Childhood_Inclusion

Earls, M. F., Andrews, J. E., & Hay, S. S. (2009). Longitudinal study of developmental and behavioral screening and referral in North Carolina's Assuring Better Child Health and Development participating practices. *Clinical Pediatrics, 48,* 824–833.

Early Childhood Comprehensive Systems Initiative. (n.d.). Retrieved from http://eccs.hrsa.gov

Early Childhood Learning and Knowledge Center. (2000). *Practicing the Collaborative Process.* Retrieved from http://eclkc.ohs.acf.hhs.gov/hslc/Family%20and%20Community%20Partnerships/Community%20Partnership/Building%20&%20Planning%20Partnerships/famcom_fts_00132_081905.html

Epps, S., & Jackson, B. (2000). *Empowered families, successful children: Early intervention programs that work.* Washington, DC: American Psychological Association.

Forrester, J. W. (1969). *Principles of system.* Cambridge, MA: Wright-Allen Press.

Foster-Fishman, P. G., & Behrens, T. R. (2007). Systems change reborn: Rethinking our theories, methods and efforts in human services reform and community-based change. *American Journal of Community Psychology, 39,* 191–196.

Foster-Fishman, P. G., Nowell, B., & Yang, H. (2007). Putting the system back into systems change: A framework for understanding and changing organizational and community systems. *American Journal of Community Psychology, 39,* 197–215.

Harbin, G., & Van Horn, J. (1990). Interagency coordinating council roles and responsibilities, Policy Alert (P.L. 99-457, Part H). Chapel Hill: Carolina Policy Studies Program, University of North Carolina. ERIC ED357578

Horwitz, S. M., Owens, P., & Simms, M. D. (2000). Specialized assessments for children in foster care. *Pediatrics, 106,* 59–66.

Hurlburt, M., Leslie, L., Landsverk, J., Barth, R. P., Burns, B. J., Gibbons, R. D., et al. (2004). Contextual predictors of mental health service use among children open to child welfare. *Archives General Psychiatry, 61,* 1217–1224.

Individuals with Disabilities Education Improvement Act (IDEIA; P.L. 108-446). (2004). Retrieved from http://www.copyright.gov/legislation/pl108-446.pdf

Johnson, L. J., Zorn, D., Kai Yung Tam, B., LaMontagne, M., & Johnson, S. A. (2003). Stakeholders' view of factors that impact successful interagency collaboration. *Exceptional Children, 69,* 195–209.

Keeping Children and Families Safe Act (P.L. 108-36). (2003). Retrieved from http://www.acf.hhs.gov/programs/cb/laws_policies/policy/im/2003/im0304a.pdf

Knitzer, J. (1997). Service integration for children and families: Lessons and questions. In R. J. Illback, C. T. Cobb, & H. M. Joseph (Eds.), *Integrated services for children and families: Opportunities for psychological practice* (pp. 3–21). Washington, DC: American Psychological Association.

Kochanek, T., & Buka, S. (1998).Patterns of service utilization: Child, maternal, and service provider factors. *Journal of Early Intervention, 21,* 217–231.

Kysor, D. F. (1995). Child and adolescent service system program: A multi-systems approach to service delivery for students with mental health needs. ERIC Doc ED386002

Lannon, C. M., Flower, K., Duncan, P., Moore, K. S., Stuart, J., & Bassewitz, J. (2008). The Bright Futures Training Intervention Project: Implementing systems to support preventive and developmental services in practice. *Pediatrics, 122,* 163–171.

Lavigne, J. V., Arend, R., Rosenbaum, D., Binns, H. J., Christoffel, K. K., Burns, A., et al. (1998). Mental health service use among young children receiving pediatric primary care. *Journal of the American Academy of Child and Adolescent Psychiatry, 37,* 1175–1183.

Leslie, L. K., Gordon, J. N., Lambros, K., Premji, K., Peoples, J., & Gist, K. (2005). Addressing the developmental and mental health needs of young children in foster care. *Developmental and Behavioral Pediatrics, 26,* 140–151.

Lewin Group. (2007). State maternal and child health early childhood comprehensive systems grant program (ECCS): Year one evaluation final report. Washington, DC: Health Resources and Services Administration, Maternal and Child Health Bureau.

Mahoney, G., & Filer, J. (1996). How responsive is early intervention to the priorities and needs of families? *Topics in Early Childhood Special Education, 16,* 437–457.

Maternal and Child Health Bureau. (2000). *Understanding Title V of the Social Security Act: A guide to the provisions of the Maternal and Child Health Block Grant.* Washington, DC: U.S. Department of Health and Human Services, Health Resources and Services Administration, Maternal and Child Health Bureau.

National Association of Social Workers. (2003). *Keeping Children and Families Safe Act of 2003*. Retrieved from http://www.socialworkers.org/advocacy/updates/2003/030503.asp

National Center for Education in Maternal and Child Health, Georgetown University. (2008). *Bright Futures*. Retrieved from http://www.brightfutures.org

National Institute for Health Care Management. (2009). *Strategies to support the integration of mental health into pediatric primary care*. Retrieved from http://nihcm.org/pdf/PediatricMH-FINAL.pdf

Newton, R. R., Litrownik, A. J., & Landsverk, J. A. (2000). Children and youth in foster care: disentangling the relationship between problem behaviors and number of placements. *Child Abuse and Neglect, 24*, 1363–1374.

Nolan, K. W., Young, E. C., Herbert, E. B., & Wilding, G. E. (2005). Service coordination for children with complex healthcare needs in an early intervention program. *Infants and Young Children, 18*, 161–170.

Office of Head Start. (2007). *Head Start State Collaboration Offices: 2007 Annual State Profiles*. Washington, DC: Department of Health and Human Services. Retrieved from http://eclkc.ohs.acf.hhs.gov/hslc/Head%20Start%20Program/State%20collaboration/HSSCO/HSSCO_2007_Profiles1%5B1%5D.pdf

Peterson, N. L. (1991). Interagency collaboration under Part H: The key to comprehensive, multidisciplinary, coordinated infant/toddler intervention services. *Journal of Early Intervention, 15*, 89–105.

Pires, S. (2008). *Building systems of care: A primer for child welfare*. Washington, DC: National Technical Assistance Center for Children's Mental Health, Georgetown University Center for Child and Human Development, Georgetown University. Retrieved from http://gucchd.georgetown.edu/72382.html

Roberts, R. N., & Wasik, B. H. (1996). Evaluating the 1992 and 1993 community integrated service systems projects. *New Directions for Evaluations, 69*, 35–49.

Rouse, H. L., & Fantuzzo, J. W. (2009). Multiple risks and educational well being: A population-based investigation of threats to early school success. *Early Childhood Research Quarterly, 24*, 1–14.

Sedlak, A. J., & Boadhurst, D. D. (1996). *The Third National Incidence Study of Child Abuse and Neglect*. Washington, DC: U.S. Department of Health and Human Services, Administration for Children, Youth, and Families.

Shelton, T. L., & Stepanek, J. S. (1994). *Family-centered care for children needing specialized health and developmental services*. Bethesda, MD: Association for the Care of Children's health. ERIC ED 381926.

Sloper, P. (2004). Facilitators and barriers for coordinated multi-agency services. *Child: Care, Health and Development, 30*, 571–580.

Smucker, K. S., Kauffman, J. M., & Ball, D. W. (1996). School-related problems of special education foster-care students with emotional or behavioral disorders: a comparison to other groups. *Journal of Emotional and Behavioral Disorders, 4*, 30–39.

Sontag, J. C., & Schacht, R. (1994). An ethnic comparison of parent participation and information needs in early intervention. *Exceptional Children, 60*, 422–433.

Stephens, R. L., Connor, T., Nguyen, H., Holden, E. W., Greenbaum, P. E., & Foster, E. M. (2005). The longitudinal comparison study of the national evaluation of the Comprehensive Community Mental Health Services for Children and their Families Program. In M. Epstein, K. Kutash, & A. Duchnowski (Eds.), *Outcomes for children and youth with behavioral and emotional disorders and their families: Programs and evaluation best practices* (pp. 525–550). Austin, TX: PRO-ED.

Stephens, R. L., Holden, E. W., & Hernandez, M. (2004). System of care practice review scores as predictors of behavioral symptomatology. *Journal of Child and Family Studies, 13,* 179–191.

Szilagyi, M. (2009). Children with special health care needs in foster care in the United States. In C. Burns (Ed.), *Disabled children living away from home in foster care and residential settings* (pp. 114–121). London: Mac Keith Press.

Taussig, H. N. (2002). Risk behaviors in maltreated youth placed in foster care: a longitudinal study of protective and vulnerability factors. *Child Abuse and Neglect, 26,* 1179–1199.

Tebes, J. K., Bowler, S. M., Shah, S., Connell, S. M., Ross, E., Simmons, R., et al. (2005). Service access and service system development in a children's behavioral health system of care. *Evaluation and Program Planning, 28,* 151–160.

Vermont Agency of Human Services. (2005). *Supporting children with disabilities and their families: An interagency agreement among early care, health and education programs and agencies in Vermont.* Retrieved from http://www.eric.ed.gov/PDFS/ED486542.pdf

Walrath, C. M., Ybarra, M. L., & Holdern, E. W. (2006). Understanding the pre-referral factors associated with differential outcomes among children receiving systems-of-care services. *Psychological Services, 3,* 35–50.

Woolverton, M. (2002). *Meeting the health care needs of children in the foster care system: Strategies for implementation.* Washington, DC: Georgetown University Child Development Center. Retrieved from http://gucchd.georgetown.edu/products/FCStrategies.pdf

Zero to Three. (2009). *Putting the pieces together for infants and toddlers: Comprehensive, coordinated systems.* Retrieved from http://www.zerotothree.org/site/DocServer/SystemsSinglesMarch5.pdf?docID=7903

Zima, B. T., Bussing, R., Freeman, S., Yang, X., Belin, T. R., & Forness, S. R. (2000). Behavior problems, academic skill delays and school failure among school-aged children in foster care: Their relationship to placement characteristics. *Journal of Child and Family Studies, 9,* 87–103.

About the Editor and Contributors

EDITOR

Louise A. Kaczmarek, PhD, is Associate Professor of Special Education and Coordinator of the Early Intervention and Early Childhood Education Programs in the School of Education at the University of Pittsburgh. She has been an active participant in training personnel in multiple discipline as part of the UCLID Center for Individuals with Disabilities at the University of Pittsburgh, a LEND grant that supports interdisciplinary leadership training. Her research has focused on the provision of support to families whose children are served in classroom-based early intervention programs, interdisciplinary training of personnel, and classroom-based language intervention strategies. Her accomplishments include principal investigator or co-principal investigator on many federally funded research, in-service training, model demonstration, and personnel preparation projects; author and co-author of numerous journal articles and book chapters; co-author of a book on social-communication interventions; and presenter at numerous conferences and in-service workshops. Dr. Kaczmarek is an associate editor of the Journal of Early Intervention (JEI).

CONTRIBUTORS

Stephen J. Bagnato, EdD, NCSP, is a Professor of Pediatrics and Psychology at the University of Pittsburgh School of Medicine and a faculty member in the Applied Developmental Psychology Program in the School of Education. Dr. Bagnato is Director of Early Childhood Partnerships (ECP) at Pitt and Children's Hospital of Pittsburgh of UPMC. In over 30 years of research, Dr. Bagnato has specialized in authentic curriculum-based assessment and program evaluation research strategies for young children at developmental risk and with neurodevelopmental disabilities in early childhood intervention programs. He has published 130 research articles, publications, and seven books in this specialty. His latest companion texts are *Authentic Assessment for Early Childhood Intervention: Best Practices* (2007), and *LINKing Authentic Assessment and Early Childhood Intervention: Best Measures for Best Practices* (2010).

LeeMarie A. Benshoff is a graduate student in the School of Education at the University of North Carolina at Chapel Hill and is working on the Recognition and Response Project (R&R). R&R is being developed at the Frank Porter Graham Child Development Institute, University of North Carolina. R&R is a tiered model for prekindergarten based on Response to Intervention (RtI), designed to provide high-quality instruction and targeted interventions that are matched to children's learning needs.

Virginia Buysse is a Senior Scientist at the Frank Porter Graham Child Development Center at the University of North Carolina at Chapel Hill. She directs a program of research on Recognition & Response (R&R), a model of Response to Intervention (RtI) for prekindergarten, funded by the Emily Hall Tremaine Foundation and the Institute for Education Sciences, U.S. Department of Education. She serves as Co-Principal Investigator on the Center for Early Care and Education Research for Dual Language Learners funded by the Office of Planning, Research, and Evaluation, Administration for Children and Families, U.S. Department of Health and Human Services; and Co-Principal Investigator on the National Professional Development Center on Inclusion and CONNECT (Center to Mobilize Early Childhood Knowledge), both funded by the Office of Special Education Programs, U.S. Department of Education. She is Past President-Elect of the *Division of Early Childhood* (DEC) of the *Council for Exceptional Children* (CEC).

Crystal Crowe is a doctoral student at the University of Florida in Gainesville. Her major area of doctoral study is early childhood special education, with emphases in early childhood policy and research methods. Ms. Crowe completed her M.Ed. in community counseling at Vanderbilt University. She has been an interventionist in early language research projects as well as a coach to parents and Head Start teachers. Currently, Ms. Crowe is involved in an interagency initiative to develop a cross-sector plan for early childhood professional development in Florida. In addition, she is a research assistant on the Embedded Instruction for Early Learning Project funded by the Institute of Education Sciences at the University of Florida.

Amy G. Dell, PhD, is a Professor and Chairperson of the Department of Special Education, Language and Literacy at the College of New Jersey. For 11 years she directed the Adaptive Technology Center for New Jersey Colleges and is now the director of the Center on Assistive Technology and Inclusive Education Studies. Dr. Dell is coauthor of the book *Assistive Technology in the Classroom: Enhancing the School Experiences of Students with Disabilities.*

Maria K. Denney, PhD, is an Assistant Professor in the School of Special Education, School Psychology and Early Childhood Studies in the College of Education at the University of Florida. She received her PhD in education with an emphasis in special education, disability, and risk studies from the University of California, Santa Barbara (UCSB) in 2003. Dr. Denney holds an MA in education with an emphasis in child and adolescent development and a BA in Spanish from UCSB. Her teaching and research interests build directly from over a decade of work with families and children at risk or with established disabilities in early intervention settings. Dr. Denney's research focuses on multicultural and linguistic issues in early childhood special education; families and disabilities; child development, disability, and poverty; integration of early intervention service delivery systems; and preservice and in-service professional development among early childhood professionals.

Cristian M. Dogaru is a pediatrician from Romania, with a PhD in child development from Oregon State University. His research is focused on children with special needs (medical and developmental). Presently he works as a Research Fellow at the Institute of Social and Preventive Medicine, University of Bern, Switzerland.

Marisa Macy, PhD, is an Assistant Professor of Education at Lycoming College. Dr. Macy conducts research in assessment, intervention, and personnel preparation. She serves on two special education editorial boards. She has received grants for both research and personnel preparation and a fellowship at the National Institute on Disability and Rehabilitation Research. Her awards for research on assessment include one from the American Education Research Association.

Susan M. Moore, JD, MA-SLP, CCC, is a Clinical Professor and the Director of Clinical Education and Services for the Department of Speech, Language and Hearing Science at the University of Colorado, Boulder. Her publications include articles and chapters focused on working with culturally and linguistically diverse children and families, early language, and literacy learning. She has collaborated with the Denver Public Schools in the Early Reading First project to help culturally diverse children. Dr. Moore is an ASHA (American Speech-Language-Hearing Association) Fellow and holds Specialty Recognition in Child Language.

Deborah A. Newton, EdD, is Associate Professor and Chairperson of the Special Education and Reading Department at Southern Connecticut State University. Dr. Newton's areas of expertise are assistive technology for education and assistive technology for computer access. She is president of the Technology and Media Division (TAM) of the Council for Exceptional Children, and she is coauthor of the textbook *Assistive Technology in the Classroom: Enhancing* the *School Experiences of Students with Disabilities.*

Cathleen Pasia is a doctoral student in School Psychology at the University of Florida. She is specializing in early childhood studies. She is a research assistant on the Embedded Instruction for Early Learning Project under the direction of Dr. Patricia Snyder.

Ellen Peisner-Feinberg, PhD, is a Senior Scientist at the Frank Porter Graham (FPG) Child Development Institute and Research Associate Professor in the School of Education at the University of North Carolina at Chapel Hill. She is leading a line of research on Recognition & Response (R&R), a model of Response to Intervention (RtI) for prekindergarten funded by the Emily Hall Tremaine Foundation and the Institute for Education Sciences, U.S. Department of Education. Dr. Peisner-Feinberg has wide experience in the study of early care and education programs, including directing the statewide evaluation of North Carolina's More at Four Prekindergarten Program since its inception and serving as a Principal Investigator on the Cost, Quality, and Child Outcomes in Child Care Centers Project, a seminal study of child care in the United States. Other current efforts include serving as a Co-Principal Investigator on the Center for Early Care and Education Research for Dual Language Learners (CECER-DLL) funded by the Office of Planning, Research, and Evaluation, Administration for

Children and Families, U.S. Department of Health and Human Services, as well as on a study of child care utilization patterns for Latino families funded by the Child Care Bureau, U.S. Department of Health and Human Services, and an evaluation of a preschool language and literacy intervention funded by the U.S. Department of Education.

Clara Pérez-Méndez, Founder and Director of Puentes Culturales, was born in Mexico and has lived in the United States since 1975. Clara is an educator, nationally recognized speaker, and consultant focused on building understanding and competence for those in education who work with linguistically diverse children and families. She is a regular lecturer in both pre-service and in-service programs preparing personnel to work with culturally diverse populations. Her involvement and expertise in early education include coordination of a bilingual early Child Find assessment team; consultation and workshop development with the Colorado Department of Education for training cultural mediators, interpreters, and translators; and collaboration with the University of Colorado at Boulder developing El Grupo de Familias (http://www.puentesculturales.com). Ms. Pérez-Méndez has a wealth of experience working with families from traditionally underrepresented backgrounds, especially Spanish-speaking families.

Jerry G. Petroff, PhD, is Associate Professor of Special Education at the College of New Jersey, where he has been teaching since 2001. Dr. Petroff's research interests include transition to postsecondary life for students with severe disabilities, early communication, and family life. Dr. Petroff is the Director of the New Jersey Consortium on Deaf Blindness (NJCDB), a community of family members, professionals, and others interested in promoting quality education for children and youth who are deaf-blind. Dr. Petroff is coauthor with Amy Dell and Deborah Newton of the book *Assistive Technology in the Classroom: Enhancing the School Experiences of Students with Disabilities*.

Kristie Pretti-Frontczak, PhD, is Professor of Early Childhood Intervention at Kent State University. She has written extensively on the topic of authentic assessment and is a coauthor on *LINKing Authentic Assessment and Early Childhood Intervention: Best Measures for Best Practices and Assessing Young Children in Inclusive Settings: The Blended Practices Approach*. She specializes in effective approaches to working with young children in inclusive settings (specifically regarding the implementation and evaluation of curriculum frameworks), and most recently on the application of Response to Intervention principles to early childhood settings.

Salih Rakap, MEd, is a doctoral student in the School of Special Education, School Psychology, and Early Childhood Studies at the University of Florida. He received a MEd in early intervention at the University of Pittsburgh. His research interests include the application evidence-based early intervention strategies in preschool classrooms, personnel preparation in early childhood special education, and inclusion. He has researched opinions of general education teachers working in public elementary schools in Turkey regarding the inclusion of students with disabilities in their classrooms. Mr. Rakap has published his work in the *European Journal of Special Needs Education*. He is a Research Assistant for the Embedded Instruction for Early Learning project funded by the Institute of Education Sciences (IES).

Sharon E. Rosenkoetter, PhD, is in the College of Health and Human Sciences at Oregon State University. Dr. Rosenkoetter studies children's development from ages 0–8, including the impact of special needs. Her research has focused on prekindergarten transition planning, emergent literacy, television viewing, and personnel development. Dr. Rosenkoetter is Project Director of Early Childhood Leadership Directions, a model demonstration project, and Rural Links, a personnel preparation project, under the U.S. Department of Education. Dr. Rosenkoetter also served as Co-Principal Investigator in Project REViEW, a study of interventions to mitigate the effects of television violence, sponsored by the U.S. Department of Education.

Beth Rous, EdD, is Associate Professor of Educational Leadership Studies at the University of Kentucky. She also serves as Director of Early Childhood at the Human Development Institute at the University of Kentucky, a center for excellence in developmental disabilities, education, research, and service. Dr. Rous has conducted research and written on early childhood topics such as accountability systems, transition, and professional development. She has authored and coauthored numerous articles and book chapters related to policy in early childhood education, and early intervention.

Carol Schroeder, MS, has been providing direct services and managing programs in the early intervention and child care fields for over 30 years. She has been active in Kentucky's coordination of a personnel development system for early care and education providers and contributed to the research activities of the federally funded National Early Childhood Transition Center (NECTC). Currently, she holds the position of Early Childhood Associate Director, Human Development Institute, University of Kentucky, and directs the Training Into Practice Project, a component of Kentucky's KIDS NOW Early Childhood Initiative.

Dawn Burger Sexton is currently a preschool teacher in a public preschool in rural Kentucky. Her class includes children who are at risk because of economic factors and children with identified disabilities. Ms. Sexton is currently enrolled in a graduate program and will receive her master's degree in Interdisciplinary Early Childhood Education through the University of Kentucky (UK). While at UK, she has worked on a number of research projects, including KIDS NOW: Kentucky Invests in Developing Success NOW; Project LINK: A Partnership to Promote LINKages among Assessment, Curriculum and Outcomes; and PROJECT PLAY: Promoting Positive Learning Outcomes through an Activity Based Approach with Young Children with Severe Disabilities. She also served as an assistant for two years at the University of Kentucky Laboratory School. Her research focuses on authentic assessment as used in a preschool setting.

Patricia A. Snyder, PhD, is the David Lawrence Jr. Endowed Chair in Early Childhood Studies and a Professor in the School of Special Education, School Psychology, and Early Childhood Studies and the Department of Pediatrics at the University of Florida. She was founder and Director of the interdisciplinary Early Intervention Institute at the Louisiana State University Health Sciences Center and has held faculty appointments at LSU Health Sciences Center, Vanderbilt University Medical Center, and Peabody College at Vanderbilt University. She has been a recipient of the Alan A. Copping Excellence in Teaching Award from the Louisiana State University system, the Merle B. Karnes Award for Service to the Division for Early Childhood (Council for Exceptional Children), the Article of the Year Award from the American Psychological Association (APA) Division 16, and a Service to the Profession award from the American Occupational Therapy Association. Dr. Snyder served from 2002 to 2007 as the editor of the *Journal of Early Intervention*. Her research focuses on the developmental impacts of early experiences and learning, social-emotional foundations for early learning, and ways families and practitioners support young children's development and learning. She has been engaged in interdisciplinary professional development activities for over 25 years. Dr. Snyder currently serves as the principal investigator for a study funded by the Institute of Education Sciences focused on examining the impacts of professional development practices on preschool teachers' use of embedded-instruction practices.

Elena P. Soukaku, DPhil, is a Postdoctoral Research Fellow at the Frank Porter Graham Child Development Institute, University of North Carolina. She is part of the team that is evaluating the results of the Recognition and Response Project (R&R), a prekindergarten high-quality instruction program. Her research interests include the quality of classroom practices in inclusive and special education settings, the effectiveness of early educational assessment and interventions, and the social and emotional development of young children. Dr. Soukakou received an American Educational Research Association (AERA) Dissertation Award in 2009.

Dale Walker, PhD, is Associate Research Professor at the Schiefelbusch Institute for Life Span Studies at the University of Kansas Juniper Gardens Children's Project and courtesy faculty in the Departments of Special Education and Applied Behavioral Science. Her research has focused on identifying the effects of early experience on language development and school readiness and developing and testing the use of meaningful outcome measures to inform intervention for infants and toddlers. She recently completed a longitudinal study of the effectiveness of interventions to promote the communication of infants and toddlers and directs a Model Demonstration Center for Promoting Language and Literacy Readiness in Early Childhood with infants and toddlers with disabilities. Dr. Walker has served as the Research Chairperson for the Division for Early Childhood, Past President of the Kansas chapter, and is a member of the State Interagency Council to advise early childhood work in Kansas. She is an associate editor of the *Journal of Early Intervention* and consulting editor for *Early Childhood Research Quarterly, Topics in Early Childhood Special Education and Young Exceptional Children Monographs*.

Advisory Board

Heidi M. Feldman, MD, PhD, is the Ballinger-Swindles Endowed Professor of Developmental and Behavioral Pediatrics at Stanford University School of Medicine. She also serves as the Medical Director of the Developmental and Behavior Pediatric Programs at Lucile Packard Children's Hospital. Dr. Feldman received her BA in Psychology (1970), summa cum laude, and her PhD in Developmental Psychology (1975) from the University of Pennsylvania. She received her MD from the University of California, San Diego (1979). Dr. Feldman has memberships in several professional societies such as the Society for Research in Child Development, the Society for Pediatric Research, and the American Academy of Pediatrics. She has served as President at the Society for the Developmental Behavioral Pediatrics. Her research focuses on developmental-behavioral pediatrics, language development in young children, and language and cognition after prematurity. She has published more than 50 peer-reviewed articles in journals like the *New England Journal of Medicine, Science, Brain and Language, Child Development, Journal of Behavioral Developmental Pediatrics, Developmental Neuropsychology,* and *Pediatrics.* She is one of the editors of the current edition of the premier textbook in her field, *Developmental-Behavioral Pediatrics* (4th ed.), published in 2009. She has served as grant reviewer for the National Institutes of Health (1992–1997 and 2008–2012) and an abstract reviewer for the Pediatric Academic Societies. Dr. Feldman has held several academic appointments: Professor at the Medical Center Line, Stanford University (2006 to present), Professor in Pediatrics, University of Pittsburgh (2000–2006), and Faculty Member at the Center for the Neural Bases of Cognition at the University of Pittsburgh/Carnegie Mellon University (2003–2006). Dr. Feldman has received several awards such as Best Doctors in America (2007–2008 and 2009–2010), Academy of Master Educators, University of Pittsburgh School of Medicine (2006),

Outstanding Alumna, University of California San Diego (2003), Ronald L. and Patricia M. Violi Professor of Pediatrics and Child Development, University of Pittsburgh (2001–2006), Excellence in Education Award, University of Pittsburgh School of Medicine (2000), and the Chancellor's Distinguished Teaching Award (1999).

Marilou Hyson, PhD, is a consultant in early child development and education and an Affiliate Faculty member in Applied Developmental Psychology at George Mason University. Formerly Associate Executive Director and Senior Consultant with the National Association for the Education of Young Children (NAEYC), Marilou contributed to the development of many position statements on issues including early learning standards, professional preparation standards, early childhood mathematics, and curriculum/assessment/program evaluation. She is the author of the recent book *Enthusiastic and Engaged Learners: Approaches to Learning in the Early Childhood Classroom*, published by NAEYC and Teachers College Press. Two book chapters on early childhood professional development and higher education systems were published in 2010. Internationally, Marilou consults in Indonesia, Bangladesh, Bhutan, and Vietnam through the World Bank and Save the Children. In the United States, Marilou consults with organizations including the Families and Work Institute, the Finance Project, the National Center for Children in Poverty, and the Society for Research in Child Development. Prior to joining NAEYC, Marilou was an SRCD Fellow in the U.S. Department of Education and Professor and Chair of the University of Delaware's Department of Individual and Family Studies. The former editor-in-chief of *Early Childhood Research Quarterly*, Marilou's research and publications have emphasized young children's emotional development, parents' and teachers' beliefs and educational practices, issues in linking research with policy and practice, and early childhood teacher preparation.

Robert Silverstein, JD, is a principal in the law firm of Powers Pyles Sutter & Verville, P.C., and he also serves as the director of the Center for the Study and Advancement of Disability Policy. Mr. Silverstein received his BS in economics, cum laude, from the Wharton School, University of Pennsylvania in 1971. He received his JD in 1974 from Georgetown University Law Center. His main areas of interest are public policy issues and the policymaking process focusing in the areas of disability, health care, rehabilitation, employment, education, social security, and civil rights. In his capacity as staff director and chief counsel to the U.S. Senate Subcommittee on Disability Policy and other positions (1986–1997), Mr. Silverstein was the behind-the-scenes architect of more than 20 bills enacted into law, including the Americans with Disabilities Act (ADA), Rehabilitation Act (1992 Amendments), the Early Intervention Program for Infants and Toddlers with Disabilities (1986), and the Individuals with Disabilities Education Act Amendments (1991, 1997 Amendments). He has presented keynotes speeches before national and state organizations and trained leaders and others in more than 40 states regarding various public policy issues and the police making process. He has more than 75 papers, articles and policy briefs on public policy issues from a disability perspective published in journals such as *Behavioral Sciences and the Law, and Iowa Law Review*. Mr. Silverstein has assisted federal, state, and local policymakers and key stakeholder groups to translate research into consensus public policy solutions addressing identified needs.

Sue Swenson is an experienced nonprofit and government leader in the field of advocacy and support for people with developmental disabilities and their families. She is interested in the application of modern management and marketing techniques to help public systems better know and serve the people they are intended to help, with a special interest in interdisciplinary applications and international collaborative efforts. Mrs. Swenson is a frequent public speaker and enthusiastic participant in forums designed to improve the lives of citizens with disabilities. She worked for The Arc of the United States as CEO. She also served as Executive Director of Joseph P. Kennedy, Jr., Foundation. She was appointed by the Clinton White House to serve as Commissioner of the Administration on Developmental Disabilities, U.S. DHHS, and served as a Kennedy Public Policy Fellow at the U.S. Senate Subcommittee on Disability Policy. Mrs. Swenson received her AB in humanities in 1975, and an AM in humanities (1977) from the University of Chicago and an MBA from the Carlson School of Management at the University of Minnesota (1986). She has three adult sons, one of whom has developmental disabilities.

Jane E. West, PhD, currently serves as Senior Vice President for Policy, Programs, and Professional Issues at the American Association of Colleges for Teacher Education (AACTE). West has written broadly on special education, disability policy and teacher preparation. She served as the staff director for the U.S. Senate Subcommittee on Disability Policy in the early 1980s under the chairmanship of Sen. Lowell P. Weicker. She currently leads AACTE's engagement in the education policy discussion related to teacher preparation, the Elementary and Secondary Education Act and the Higher Education Act.

Index

CPSIA information can be obtained at www.ICGtesting.com
Printed in the USA
BVOW011638070213

312625BV00003B/58/P